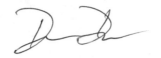

RE-THINKING PAIN

A Ground-Breaking Guide to Understanding & Healing Pain

DREW DRENTH, M.S., P.T.

The information in this book is not intended to replace the services of your current healthcare team. You are advised to consult with your physician regarding specific health concerns, in particular, those that may require diagnosis or immediate medical attention. The author takes no responsibility for any possible consequence resulting from any treatment, action, or application of medicine, to any person reading or following the information from this book.

Printed in the United States of America by Morris Publishing
3212 East Highway 30, Kearney, NE 68847

Library of Congress Control Number: 2006909396
ISBN: 978-0-9792168-0-0

Additional copies of this book may be purchased online at:
www.rethinkpain.com

ACKNOWLEDGEMENTS

I'd like to express my heartfelt gratitude to everyone who contributed to this project. In particular, to Ted Troxell for his invaluable roles of wordsmith, editor, and convivial traveler in the world of ideas; Debra Noë and Kim Pickler for their helpful comments and suggestions; fellow physical therapists David Butler and Barrett Dorko for their thought-provoking writings; and my wonderful wife, Jenna, and our three children, for their ongoing love and support.

"No form of illiteracy in the U.S. is more widespread or costly than ignorance about pain."

—David Morris, *Illness and Culture in the Postmodern Age*

CONTENTS

PREFACE

Throughout my graduate training in physical therapy, I was taught that pain resulted from a host of bodily dysfunctions: stuck joints, slipped discs, torn tendons, tight muscles, and the like. Proceeding under this assumption, little emphasis was placed on studying pain as an independent subject. In fact, though I did not recognize it at the time, my physical therapy training was not wholly unlike that of a mechanic. This was exemplified in its emphasis on the analysis of "body mechanics" with respect to pain. The subjective, or what could be called the "interior" aspects of pain, were not thought to be as relevant.

Like any professional eventually comes to understand, the neatly packaged explanations offered in the academy often disintegrate when faced with the messy peculiarities of human experience. For me, this came to a head while taking my third clinical rotation, stationed in an outpatient therapy clinic in Michigan. While there, I became confused and frustrated with the inconsistent results I was witnessing from one patient to another. I wondered why some people recovered from painful conditions so quickly, while for others, nothing seemed to work.

As is the case in many training situations, I received the standard consolation for mediocre outcomes. "Things will get better," I was told, "as soon as you get more experience under your belt." But as I carefully observed my instructors, I noticed that their patients did not always respond with consistency and predictability, even continuing to report pain and dysfunction after weeks of intensive treatment.

Since my years as a student, I have continued to wrestle practically and intellectually with the complexities and intricacies of pain. In doing so, I began to recognize the need for a new paradigm, a new way of conceptualizing pain. Through extensive observation, study, and experimentation, it became clear to me that pain could not be accurately explained as a simple product of bodily damage or abnormalities. Instead, understanding pain often required a consideration of factors beyond human anatomy: things like stress, expectations, emotions, and tension. It seemed necessary to start thinking of pain in terms of both body and mind—sometimes just called the "bodymind." To help my patients, I needed a way to think about pain that went beyond mechanical views of the body.

At first, I approached this notion of the bodymind theoretically, primarily through reading and brainstorming about its workings. In fact, it was not long before I thought I had much of it figured out and penned the first draft of this book. While doing so, however, I realized that there were still some missing pieces.

One of these pieces involved an important connection between pain and bodily tension. Since I had been aware of persistent muscle tension in my neck since I was in high school, I knew that I had a task in front of me: I would need to unpack my own tension before I could come to grips with the question of pain. As a physical therapist, I had already studied the body from the outside, now, as a student of the bodymind, I would need to do so from the inside.

As I began my explorations, I did not anticipate the can of worms I was opening. Up to that point, I had been living in a mental world that was largely disconnected from my body and its processes. I labored under the belief that I was not my body; rather, I *had* a body. My tension, therefore, was something external to my mind, coming from that thing called my body. It was like my body had a mind of its own and I was left with little say in the matter.

The more I began to explore, however—working with my breathing, observing my muscle tension, experimenting with different movements and postures—the more I realized that I could actually influence my bodily affairs, including my resting levels of tension. My mind and body were not separate agents at war with each other, but comprised an integrated whole.

Approaching pain from an integrated bodymind perspective has been invaluable to me personally, as well as my patients. Though certainly not the last word on pain, I am confident that this book can nudge us in a better direction, toward a more honest and comprehensive understanding of this challenging topic. I hope that you will join me on this exciting journey of *Re-Thinking Pain*.

INTRODUCTION

The human quest for understanding and alleviating pain is not a recent one, as indicated by early historical records.[1] By its very nature, pain quickly captures our attention, beckoning us to investigate its potential causes, as well as how its demands might be satisfied. Pain is now the most frequently asserted medical complaint, affecting the lives of more than 50 million Americans annually.[2] In fact, many researchers now view pain as an epidemic.

Despite ongoing advancements in medical technology, it is not unusual for those experiencing chronic pain to derive little long-term benefit from a gamut of diagnostic tests and procedures. This inconsistent relationship between technology and the prevalence of chronic pain has prompted both physicians and patients to scratch their heads in bewilderment. Broken bones or blocked arteries can be diagnosed with a machine, pain cannot. Instead, healthcare professionals must rely on a person's self-report regarding his or her experience of pain. Often, patients get the implicit or explicit message that there is no "objective basis" for their pain, which may leave them feeling that their experience is somehow invalid or illegitimate. This, of course, only exacerbates the problem. Perhaps, you (or someone you know) have experienced this first hand.

In conjunction with the inherent difficulty of understanding pain through the use of medical tests, pain may also resist prediction and control. For many people, pain feels chaotic and random, striking when least expected. Pain's insidious nature can engender frustration, foiling our plans for controlling our lives and circumstances.

Pain is also notorious for disrupting daily affairs. Since it is capable of commanding our utmost attention and hijacking our consciousness, persistent pain can make it difficult to effectively attend to anything else. In some instances, pain can be all-consuming, usurping physical, mental, and emotional energies. Though other types of illness can hinder day-to-day functioning, most pale in comparison to the pernicious effects of chronic pain.

As a result of its dismantling effects on daily life, it comes as no surprise that chronic pain is frequently coupled with disability, depression, and lost time from work. Moreover, the reverberating effects of chronic pain are not confined to the individual, but inevitably infiltrate families, relationships, work life, the community, and ultimately, society. So a painful condition is never merely a personal concern, but also a social one. Unfortunately, the social ramifications of pain, recognized by most cultures throughout history, have been largely neglected in our modern healthcare system.

Since pain is both a bodily and social problem, any serious attempt to understand it must assume a holistic approach. Unfortunately, the word "holistic" often carries New Age connotations which serve to obscure its essential meaning of "whole" or "complete." For clarification, when I speak of approaching pain holistically, I am referring to its physical, mental, emotional, and sociocultural aspects. It is my fervent belief that the epidemic prevalence of pain in our society is largely a result of our failure to consider this bigger picture.

Considering Pain in Context

Viewing pain holistically asks that we attend to its context, as it is the context of pain that often determines its expression and intensity. The importance of context can be conveyed through a variety of anecdotes.

Many accounts tell of soldiers feeling little or no pain after incurring battle wounds if they know they will soon be returning home. Similarly, athletes experiencing injury during a sporting event are often able to continue competing, relatively unhindered by pain. In India, men engage in tribal rituals involving swinging from large hooks sunk into the muscles of their backs and experience no pain.[3] From such examples, it is evident that physical injury is no guarantee of pain. Rather, the nature of a person's experience, painful or otherwise, depends significantly on contextual factors.

If these reports of painless injuries are a bit odd, their opposite is perhaps even stranger: the presence of pain in absence of injury. For instance, amputees frequently report experiencing pain in the portion of the limb that was removed many years prior. This is usually referred to as phantom pain, which is not intended to mean that the pain is not real, but that the area in which the pain is experienced is no longer physically present.

As another example, a study completed by the Baylor College of Medicine involved 100 paid volunteers who were told that an electric stimulator might produce a headache. What the subjects did not know was that the stimulator would generate nothing more than a low humming sound. Despite this, the results indicated that nearly *half* of the volunteers reported pain.[4]

The strange behavior of pain beckons us to consider its contexts. Our bodies are not adequately understood as isolated pain factories, but are nested within contexts that involve past experiences, meaning, values, beliefs, expectations, emotions, neuromuscular responses, etc. Just as we act on our environments, so too are we influenced by our life contexts at every step.

As I will reiterate frequently, the fact that pain is a holistic and context-dependent phenomena is actually good news if you struggle with chronic or recurrent pain. After all, if chronic pain results exclusively from bodily damage, there would seem to be little you could do to personally affect it. On the other hand, if your pain is influenced by factors that are modifiable, you can work to implement changes and regain a sense of control over your experience.

The Debate over Pain

In both academic and applied fields, disagreement persists as to the best way to approach chronic pain. Some people believe that a cure should be sought in every instance, while others feel that chronic pain is not amenable to being cured and, therefore, treatment should focus on coping strategies rather than trying to eliminate the pain. I see this debate as not particularly useful for a couple reasons:

First, people throughout history have recovered from of a variety of illnesses which at the time were deemed intractable, including those involving pain. It is therefore presumptuous, perhaps even unethical, for anyone to proclaim that recovery from chronic pain is impossible. By the same token, research and experience does seem to indicate that the longer a painful problem exists, the more difficult it becomes to fully recover. Since recovery depends largely on the individual, it is understandably difficult for clinicians to offer an accurate prognosis with respect to chronic pain.

I also challenge the assumption among some pain researchers that pain management strategies can serve to improve function but are unlikely to significantly reduce pain. This is a rather limiting argument, akin to suggesting that exercise can make you body stronger but will not make you feel any better. Such sentiments seem to lack respect for the human organism as a unified entity, in which even small changes carry the potential to powerfully alter the experience of the whole.

About this Book

This book is intended for general readership as well as healthcare professionals. In our increasingly technological society, we are conditioned to believe that problem-solving requires a high degree of specialization and technical analysis. This belief appears especially prevalent with respect to pain, as the medical and pharmaceutical communities continue to construe pain as something that needs to be measured objectively and remedied through biomedical advancements. Though technology can be useful in some instances, the vast majority of painful problems can be managed through simpler means that do not require painstaking analysis or expensive equipment.

I have found that pain can be eliminated, or at least significantly improved, through the strategies suggested in this book. Though many of these strategies may sound simple, they are not necessarily easy. We all know that habits can be hard to break, especially when pain is involved. Nonetheless, if you can embrace and apply the contents of this book, you can and will improve.

As with other books, multiple readings may be required in order to gain a solid understanding of the material. So I suggest lowering any expectations for an instantaneous cure (although this does not negate the possibility) and instead view the book as a guide to be consulted regularly over the course of your recovery. As your understanding of your own situation deepens, you will gain further insights from each successive reading.

Generally, it is my objective is to provide you with a better understanding of pain which you can readily apply to your own circumstances. More specifically, this book is intended to facilitate the following:

- *Manageable levels of pain*:   A strongpoint of this book is its capacity for application to a variety of painful conditions (see Appendix IV for a list of examples). If you are wondering if this book can remedy your pain, I suggest patiently and persistently applying its concepts to your particular situation and observing the changes. If you are like most people, you can achieve a significant reduction in pain.

- *A scientific, yet holistic understanding of pain*[5]: As indicated above, pain is largely influenced by life contexts. So it is necessary to consider not only physical factors, but the social, psychological, and emotional contexts of your pain.

- *An enhanced understanding of your bodymind*: Consistent with my own experience described in the Preface, it appears that most of us live in a divided world in which we perceive our minds as separate from our bodies. As I will describe in detail, this belies the undeniable interplay that transpires between mind and body.

The fact that body and mind are one, illustrated by use of the term "bodymind," is supported both by empirical research and common experiences. I will describe how you can harness the inherent connectedness of your bodymind to reduce pain and improve your life.

- *A restored sense of control over your reality*: It is natural for us to desire control over our lives, including our health. Research has shown that both humans and animals demonstrate greater immunity and quickened recovery from illness when a sense of control exists over their circumstances. For instance, if your physician tells you that your pain is being caused by a defect in your spine, you may come to believe that you have little opportunity for controlling your pain. In contrast, if you are informed that your pain may be related to factors that can be altered, such as those described in this book, you are more likely to experience a sense of hope and optimism. Through this book, I hope to equip you with an increased perception of control over your pain.

A Word on Format

Perhaps a bit unlike other books that involve an element of self-help, I will not be laying out a step-by-step program for you to follow. There are couple reasons for this. First, no two people are exactly alike with respect to pain; what works for you may not work the same for your friend. Moreover, since pain can be driven by a multiplex of factors, it makes little sense to approach it via a predetermined, linear format. Doing so would be like reducing a three-dimensional object by one or two dimensions.

Because of the holistic nature of our topic, the format of this book is largely categorical. I will be discussing a variety of factors that may contribute to pain, as well as different management strategies. In doing so, I grant you the freedom to determine the application of this material to your own situation. My hope is, with time, you will attain a deeper understanding of your pain, one that surpasses any surface utility associated with step-by-step approaches.

With that said, in order to provide some assistance in organizing your thoughts with respect to pain management, I offer a basic outline in the form of the acronym "CEO." I like the CEO concept because it implies that you are in charge of your health and are empowered to improve it. The following three points will be elaborated throughout this book:

Change your thoughts and behavior toward pain.

Enhance your bodily awareness.

Overhaul other aspects of your health and life.

1

NEW LENSES FOR PAIN

"We don't see the world as it is, but as we are."—William James

"Prevailing cultural orthodoxy is more powerful than any conspiracy…Orthodoxy does not have a beginning or an end, it simply is; engrained within the consciousness of each individual it goes largely unquestioned, however bizarre its consequences." —Martin J. Walker

"If there is anything our society should be doing for people with chronic illness today, it would be to help them figure out better stories to tell when their existing stories are not working."—Howard Brody

Many us believe and act as if the world is just as we perceive it to be. In other words, we view the world as pre-given rather than relative to our personal perspectives. In doing so, we forget that the world often appears differently to others.

As an example, imagine the images portrayed by two different cameras, one with high levels of resolution and another that is less precise. If the same object is captured with both cameras, will the two photos look the same? For anyone familiar with photography, the answer is clearly "no" (especially in larger prints), as the quality of the camera will influence the appearance of the object (the same could be said of high definition televisions). Now, imagine two people at a baseball game. A person who is not a baseball fan or whose favored team loses will perceive the game (especially the umpiring!) differently than a baseball lover whose team wins. Likewise, two reporters witnessing the same event will frequently produce conflicting interpretations.

The above examples point toward the fact that the lenses we use to view the world (both actually and metaphorically) influence the nature of what we apprehend; we see things as we have been conditioned to see them. Or, as the quote above puts it so eloquently: "We don't see the world as it is, *but as we are.*" Thus, what you think of as *the* world is better understood as *your* world.

What does this philosophical lesson have to do with pain? The take home point is that the influence of our personalized lenses is not limited to baseball games or political preference, but they also color how we interpret our bodily experiences—including pain. As a result, pain is different for everyone, since it is shaped by a variety of individual factors. Or, as we learned previously, it depends on context.

We will explore different factors that influence pain throughout this book, but before doing so, please take a moment to consider the following questions regarding your experience and beliefs about pain. You may wish to record your answers on a separate sheet of paper.

1. What do you believe originally caused your pain?

2. What factors do you feel continue to contribute to your pain?

3. What do you think makes your pain worse? Better?

4. Do you expect to fully recover? Why or why not?

5. What information has influenced your beliefs about your condition to this point?

Stories & Pain

Whether you realize it or not, it is likely that your responses to these questions arose from a story that you have developed about your pain experience. Stories are the preferred vessels for us to organize and interpret our experiences in a meaningful way. We tell political stories, religious stories, historical stories, family stories, cultural stories, among others. Such stories provide explanations for our ever-inquiring, pattern-seeking minds. They allow us to impose a semblance of meaning on what otherwise might feel like chaos. Stories give us direction and a sense of control over our destiny, thereby reducing uncomfortable perceptions of uncertainty about the future.

For better or worse, stories are how we negotiate life, including our experiences with pain. Stories about pain typically incorporate details regarding its perceived origins (past), its current course and meaning (present), and expectations regarding its resolution (future). Here is an example:

"I first injured my back when I was a teenager and fell off my bicycle. It seemed better for a while, but resumed hurting when I tweaked it playing basketball in college. At that point, I visited the doctor who informed me that I had a few discs that were degenerating. He told me to take it easy and stay away from strenuous physical activity. Unfortunately, I had always loved being active and his advice seemed to take the wind out of my sails. Sometime shortly after, I started to think of myself as having a permanently damaged back and decided to restrict myself to desk jobs, something I thought I would never do. Looking back, it seems that working non-physical jobs hasn't helped my back much, as I've had innumerable flare-ups over the years. At this point, I am just really frustrated. I don't feel like myself anymore. I just wish the pain would just go away. None of the treatments I've tried have provided more than temporary relief. In fact, I often find myself worrying that my back may never get any better. I'm just tired of it, that's all."

Because of the central role that such stories assume in our daily affairs, it is important for us to consider their origins. With some investigation, it is common to discover that many of our stories are not wholly original, but have incorporated the views of others. We may borrow ideas from family members, the medical community, the media, the educational system, religious authorities, etc., and assimilate them into our stories. The contents of this book, for example, cannot be divorced from what I have read, heard, and experienced over the course of my life. Just as a pot is shaped by the potter who formed it, our stories—our ways of viewing the world—are molded by the contexts in which we are (and have been) immersed. The following figure illustrates the relationship between our personal experiences, culture, and the stories we use for understanding pain.

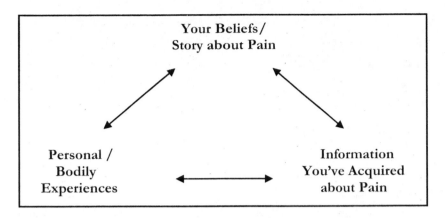

Since our stories about pain are not exempt from outside influences, particularly culture, it is imperative to examine the content of these messages. In America, we seem to think that pain is caused almost exclusively by some kind of identifiable damage to the body. This suggests that the human body is analogous to a machine, and that pain is caused by the harming or degradation its parts. The development of this belief, which I will frequently refer to as "the body-machine story," is firmly rooted in American history, as modern medical thought evolved in sync with industrial development. Thus, viewing the body and its processes in mechanical terms arose quite naturally.

The prevailing dominance of the body-machine story in American culture probably resulted from its practical simplicity, as well as its reinforcement in many of our ordinary experiences. For instance, we know that physical injuries, such as falling off a bike, tend to be painful. If we were to end up breaking an arm, we would likely experience pain, and the injury may need to be set or surgically-repaired. Since this is similar to fixing a machine, there is certainly some truth to the body-machine story. However, as with other explanations, it is frequently extended beyond its efficacy.

In our current cultural understanding, the vast majority of painful conditions have come to be interpreted in a mechanistic way. For instance, much of wrist pain is now assumed to be caused by a nerve being compressed in the wrist (i.e., carpal tunnel syndrome), heel pain by bone spurs, shoulder pain by damaged rotator cuffs, back and neck pain by disc problems, etc. You have most likely heard casual explanations like "I've got a bad back," "My body is worn-out because I've worked demanding jobs all my life," "I've got a disc out," and so on. Such accounts are rooted in the widespread body-machine story and are prevalent throughout both the medical community and the population at large.

What Difference Does a Story Make?

At this point in our discussion you may be wondering: "Does it really matter how I interpret, explain, or understand my pain? After all, I've got pain, what does this other stuff have to do with that reality?" As will become clearer as we proceed, how you understand pain in general, as well as you own situation, is critical to how you experience pain. In other words, how you think and what you believe about pain influences how you feel, and vice versa.

Although some people may suggest that beliefs are benign with respect to pain, I strongly disagree. We simply cannot escape the fact that our stories—the way we view the world and our plight—powerfully affect our behavior, emotions, and, subsequently, our health. What you believe about pain engenders certain actions and consequences, whether positive or negative. With this in mind, I offer the following proposal:

Not all stories about pain are equally beneficial (or equally accurate), and therefore, it is essential to seriously evaluate the content, validity, and implications of your story.

Throughout this book, we will learn how the predominant body-machine story is inadequate for fully understanding pain, as well as why strict adherence to such a story often serves to exacerbate pain and impede healing. It is time that we begin to see pain through new lenses, lenses broad enough to capture all of its intricate dimensions.

New Lenses for Viewing Pain

"Sometimes the best art isn't immediately obvious… But if you give it another try, it might reach you in a way you never thought possible. It's a bold move to see again, read again, and listen again."—Erin McKeown

With reference to this quote, I think what is true of art is also true of ideas. Though sometimes difficult at first, taking a new perspective on your pain can make a world of difference. The new lenses I will help you construct involve consideration of your circumstances, stress, emotions, beliefs, and other factors with respect to your pain.

The notion that mind, body, and emotions are intertwined should not seem novel or foreign to you. For instance, you may have noticed how certain thoughts or memories produce an emotional response *in your body*. Fearful memories may cause an acceleration of the heartbeat and a tensing of muscles. Sadness can engender the perception of a collapsing or heaviness in your chest, which we often call a "broken heart." We've all experienced such connections between bodily sensations and emotions, as well as their connections to our thoughts. What you may not have done to this point is incorporate these experiences into a more comprehensive understanding of your pain.

The following chapters contain the ingredients necessary to assist you in re-thinking pain in general, as well as your situation in particular. By remaining open to the new ideas and possibilities set forth in this book, your perspective on pain will broaden and deepen, opening a new world for exploring your health and well-being.

Chapter

2

Beyond the Body-Machine

"The truth is pain is a very poor reporting system."—Patrick Wall

"Backache has been common throughout recorded history, but back pain as a disabling medical condition appears to be a twentieth-century phenomenon."—Robert Gillette

"One of the most dependable occurrences in clinical care is the practitioner's inability to draw a precise one-to-one correlation between reported symptoms and disease diagnosis." —Arthur Kleinman

Stories of pain are flourishing in America, as pain is reported in approximately 80% of physician visits.[1] Despite this, many people find that their questions about the causes and recourse of their pain go unanswered. In this chapter, we will begin to explore some

17

explanations by examining important research findings. In doing so, some of these commonly asked questions will become less puzzling:

- How could the MRI indicate that nothing is wrong when I have such severe pain?

- How and why could my pain arise so suddenly, seemingly for no reason at all?

- Why is it that many people heal without treatment, while others fail to respond even to extensive treatment?

- How can two people whose spines appear similar on an MRI report completely different symptoms?

- Why do some people seem to be in pain all the time while others remain pain-free?

- Why do surgeries and medications often fail to eliminate pain and other symptoms?

Finding #1: Bodily abnormalities are inconsistent determinants of who will experience pain.

According to recent estimates, 40-90% of all doctor visits involve problems that probably cannot be diagnosed, much less treated effectively, with traditional medical treatments.[2] This is especially true for pain, as testing rarely reveals abnormalities that fully and accurately account for reported symptoms.[3] According to the authors of *Back Sense*, the incidence of serious pathology causing back pain is only about *one in two hundred.* In one study of 10,000 cases of low back pain submitted for compensation, 75% were found to have no pertinent structural abnormalities.[4] From a body-machine perspective, this evidence appears perplexing considering the epidemic proportions of Americans reporting back pain.

For those admitted to the emergency room, 37% report experiencing no pain at the time of injury.[5] Both imaging (MRI, X-ray, etc.) and cadaver studies continue to confirm that structural degeneration and other irregularities are often painless.[6] This is true of bulging discs, torn rotator cuffs, bone spurs, arthritis, cartilage damage, and a host of other "abnormalities" (see Appendix IV for a more extensive list of conditions). One example, reported by Fox and colleagues,[7] was the discovery that "large, space-occupying abnormalities" in the cervical spine often produced no symptoms whatsoever. This is underpinned by a significant amount of research showing poor correlations between spinal disc abnormalities and reported pain levels.[8]

One seven-year follow-up study of initially asymptomatic subjects concluded: "The present study demonstrated the inability of magnetic resonance scans (MRIs) to predict the development of back pain over a seven-year period."[9] As Dr. Arthur Kleinman writes, "The diagnosis of a structural or functional abnormality tells the practitioner little at all about severity of symptoms, functional abnormality, or course and treatment response."[10]

In addition to the above research, those who engage in intentional self-injuring behavior usually report experiencing no pain. In fact, inducing physical damage to their bodies seems to alleviate distress, perhaps in a way similar to the "runner's high."

Though such evidence suggests that the correlation between bodily abnormality and pain is questionable, this does not mean that the pain is imagined or that the body is uninvolved. In fact, some bodily factors which can contribute to pain, such as muscle tension, will not show up on an MRI or X-ray. The role of the body in pain will be discussed further in Chapter 5.

Finding #2: Psychological and social factors are useful predictors of who will develop pain, including chronic pain and disability.

This is supported by multiple studies,[11] including a frequently cited study conducted by Boeing Corporation that included over 3,000 of its employees.[12] In this study, the researchers began by collecting baseline data on individuals and the nature of their jobs. They proceeded to follow them over the course of four years, and witnessed nearly three hundred employees develop back pain. After analyzing the data, it was determined that initially measured psychological and social factors, such as job dissatisfaction and specific personality traits, better predicted who developed back pain than other factors, including the physical requirements of the job. Studies such as this challenge the common belief that physically demanding jobs cause pain and disability. In reality, individual *perceptions* of the job may be more critical.[13]

It is important to recognize that psychological factors also have physical correlates. When we are stressed and feel tense, that tension manifests through our muscles. That is, after all, why we *feel* the stress. Therefore, we should pause before elevating psychological factors over physical ones, remembering that we are dealing with a unified bodymind.

Finding #3: Culture influences our expectations, interpretations, and experiences of pain.

- American patients with low back pain use more medications and experience more distress and functional impairment than those from New Zealand[14] or Japan.[15]

- Americans with chronic back pain display the most dysfunction when compared to other cultures around the world.[16]

- Claims of chronic symptoms of whiplash vary widely depending on each country's compensational system.[17]

What is the overarching theme of these findings? It appears that, as described in Chapter 1, our predominant cultural story and medical system powerfully influence our beliefs, behaviors, and bodily experiences. According to Kleinman, the type of symptoms that are viewed to be concerning, as well as beliefs about treatment and recovery, vary widely among different cultures.[18] For example, those in developing nations don't view back pain as a serious problem, but as an occasional part of life. They may ambulate without shoes, sleep on dirt floors, and perform exhausting physical labor, all while rarely complaining of debilitating back pain.[19]

Contrastingly, cultures such as ours have come to view back pain as something to be feared, leading to its conception as a serious medical problem. Such beliefs have certainly contributed to our current epidemic of painful problems. In *The Back Pain Revolution*, orthopedic surgeon and researcher Dr. Gordon Waddell implicates three misguided beliefs as responsible for catalyzing the exponential increases in back pain: the belief that back pain always signifies a problem with the spine, that it is necessitated by injury, and that it should be treated with rest.

Finding #4: Common treatments for pain are characterized by inconsistent outcomes.

It is generally acknowledged that surgical intervention is only about 50% effective for significantly reducing back pain. Even in instances when pain is reduced initially, recurrence is not uncommon.[20] Moreover, for those surgeries that are effective, it is likely that patients' expectations for improvement may be largely responsible for the improvement (i.e., the "placebo effect"; see Chapter 4). The few studies that are available comparing real surgeries to sham surgeries (i.e., when patients' skin was simply cut and stitched) have shown no significant difference in post-surgical outcomes.[21] One review of surgical records found that symptom relief was obtained half of the time even though surgeons found little that needed to be repaired.[22] Non-surgical treatments for pain, such as those administered in physical therapy and chiropractic, have also failed to demonstrate consistent outcomes.[23]

Finding #5: Emotions play a significant role in pain.

Modern medicine has attempted to view pain independently of emotions and other factors. In cross-cultural studies, however, researchers have learned that the languages of many traditional cultures do not even include words for what Westerners conceptualize as "pain" (i.e., bodily pain sensations). Instead, bodily sensations remain undifferentiated from expressions of human suffering such as grief, anguish, sorrow, guilt, and shame.[24]

The emotional aspect of pain has also been verified empirically, as the brain contains pathways mutually involved in both pain and emotions.[25] This may serve to explain why psychological medications, such as anti-depressants, have been shown to reduce pain. This connection between pain and emotions will be expounded further in Chapter 7.

Concluding Thoughts

The above evidence points to our need for a new way of understanding pain. If you are struggling with pain, this is good news because it opens new possibilities for recovery. Despite the ominous-sounding diagnoses you may have received in the past, they may actually be of small significance with respect to your pain.

CHAPTER

3

THE LAST STRAW

Thus far, we have discussed the necessity of re-thinking our understanding of pain and have surveyed pertinent research findings. In this chapter, I will lay the foundation for a more comprehensive understanding of the how's and why's of pain. In particular, the concepts of balance and threshold, which assume a central position in this chapter, can be viewed as fundamental to our enterprise. My hope is that the concepts introduced here will allow you to more readily assimilate the diverse ideas and evidence presented throughout the book.

The Bodymind

For centuries, philosophers and other thoughtful folks have concerned themselves with the relationship between the mind and body. What is the mind? Is it fundamentally distinct from the body? How could a seemingly immaterial mind interface with a material body? In philosophy, these age-old questions are often situated within what is frequently called the mind-body problem.

Many people have attempted to equate the mind with the brain. Scientists continue in their attempts to read minds by measuring physiological processes in the brain with advancing technology. Though what we typically conceive as "mind" is certainly dependent on our fantastically convoluted brains, it is more than an immaculate orchestra of brain waves. In reality, intelligence and consciousness (i.e., mind) are present throughout our bodies, even down to the cellular level.[1]

Though the nuances of the mind-body problem will continue to be debated, one thing is clear: the mind and body interact and they do so at every step. Together, they form one unitary system— the bodymind. You might imagine mind and body as comprising two sides of the same coin: though they may have different qualities, they nonetheless constitute a single entity.

Understanding this mind-body connection is no longer relegated exclusively to the armchairs of philosophers, but has now become the subject of emerging fields of scientific study, including what has come to be known as "psychoneuroimmunology." In layman's terms, these researchers are interested in understanding the communication that is constantly occurring between different bodily systems, as well as relevant implications for human health. For example, Dr. Candace Pert, in her book *Molecules of Emotion*, describes her pioneering research into molecules that regulate emotion and how they may serve as intermediaries between body and mind.

Since mind and body are inherently interrelated, pain cannot be said to exist exclusively in either domain. Rather, like emotions, it is best considered an integrated bodymind phenomenon. When viewed this way, pain must be approached more broadly, as we recognize its emergence from an admixture of sensations, beliefs, emotions, concerns, and plans for trying to alleviate it.

Pain as an Indicator of Imbalance

Biologists would agree that organisms, including humans, must remain within certain boundaries in order to flourish. Survival depends on the ability of an organism to maintain balance both internally and with its surroundings, while tolerating only limited amounts of deviation.

For instance, humans cannot survive long while immersed in subzero temperatures, just as we cannot long tolerate an internal temperature surpassing 105 degrees. Generally speaking, if our bodily limits are exceeded for an extended period of time, we run the risk for serious, perhaps even fatal, consequences.

Most people are familiar with the importance of balance in life to some extent. After all, we have been told to eat a balanced diet, to moderate activity with rest, to balance work with family, etc. Moreover, our physicians describe and carefully monitor bodily signifiers of balance, such as cholesterol, blood pressure, hemoglobin, blood cells, etc.

Since life depends on balance, the bodymind must remain sensitive to deviation from it. Although balance is usually regulated outside of our conscious awareness (such as when insulin is released into the bloodstream to maintain blood sugar levels), this is not exclusively the case. I suggest that our conscious experiences[2]— sight, sound, taste, fatigue, hunger, mood changes, nausea, pain, etc.—also facilitate the restoration of balance by prompting us to behave in certain ways.

For example, if the body needs energy or nutrients, the experience of hunger promotes eating, which corrects the imbalance. This is consistent with the ideas of renowned pain researcher Patrick Wall who conceptualized pain as a "need state."[3] In other words, pain indicates the presence of imbalance, as well as the need for corrective action.

As stated above, we can tolerate a certain degree of imbalance without severe detriment. You know through experience that certain amounts of force, such as wrestling with a toddler, will not harm your body. As the force increases, however, so does the potential for harm. The point at which imbalance becomes severe enough to induce pain, I will call the pain threshold or bodymind threshold.

The Pain Threshold

If you stub your toe and experience pain, it is pretty obvious that the pain resulted from an injury to your toe. In other cases, however, the explanation is not as evident. This leads to an important question:

Why and how can pain sometimes strike
suddenly, seemingly without warning or explanation?

This is a question that I frequently encounter as a physical therapist, as my patients often wonder how excruciating pain can begin in the absence of any apparent injury. In order to understand this phenomenon, we must understand the concept of threshold.

As introduced above, the pain threshold is crossed once an imbalance reaches a certain level of severity. It is critical to recognize that this may result not only from physical injury, but also as a result of emotional, psychological, social, and/or environmental imbalances (remember: pain is context-dependent). This concept of threshold appears quite useful for understanding why pain (or other bodily conditions) may suddenly manifest:

If the bodymind is already imbalanced and near its threshold, it may only take a small alteration in balance to instigate pain. ("The straw that broke the camel's back.")

Some may find it strange that the bodymind would react so suddenly and intensely to such slight shifts in balance.[4] It is necessary to recognize, however, that what we perceive to be a sudden onset of pain is often preceded by warning signals—increasing tension, mood changes, fatigue, anxiety, etc.—that we may overlook or ignore. These warning signals are designed to promote modifications in our behavior so that balance may be restored. It follows, then, that by increasing our sensitivity and responsiveness to these preliminary signs of imbalance, we can reduce the likelihood of developing full-blown pain or illness.

I would also like to emphasize that the concepts of threshold and bodymind balance are holistic in nature. This conveys the value of looking at the balance of your life and bodymind as a whole, rather than simply thinking mechanistically about the problematic area. Moreover, it appears that improving your overall health and well-being may facilitate reconciliation of a variety of bodily ailments—including pain. To some extent then, we can understand a person's bodymind experience as a ledger of positives and negatives. If the positive side is kept strong, the likelihood of experiencing pain or illness is greatly reduced. However, if life circumstances become too stressful, the threshold is more likely to be crossed.

A Real-Life Illustration of the Pain Threshold

The threshold concept has served quite useful for understanding my wife's history of back pain. While in college, she experienced several episodes of back pain entailing multiple days of bed rest. At the time, she was uncertain as to the cause of her pain and took the familiar path of seeking out numerous specialists and undergoing multiple diagnostic tests. Despite extensive testing, little "objective" evidence was found and she was left with a few different drugs, many unanswered questions, and ongoing concerns about what she perceived as her "bad back." Not an uncommon scenario.

Since discovering that these episodes were stress-related, she has had very little back trouble over the last several years. However, this past year she had started a new job with upcoming deadlines, was feeling pressured to prepare the house for weekend visitors, was dealing with a bad cold and sick children, all while I was working fairly long days. These multiple pressures came to a head in an intense bout of back pain. Her bodymind's threshold had been broken, her system overwhelmed, and at that point, there would be no quick resolution. The pain effectively forced her to take a much needed rest break, to the tune of several days in bed.

The role of stress in onsets of acute back pain (discussed more in Chapter 6) is something that many people fail to recognize. Instances of insidious pain are often described as the "back going out" and attributed to "no reason at all" or to some physical event, such as sleeping or bending the wrong way. In light of our discussion above, however, any physical activity associated with a sudden onset of pain (outside of an obvious injury) may simply be an incidental last straw in the crossing of the bodymind's pain threshold.[5]

Final Thoughts

Though we tend to associate pain with physical injury, its scope is often much broader. In this chapter, we have discussed the fact that pain signals a state of imbalance in the bodymind. Some people may find this explanation of pain puzzling, wondering why the bodymind would use such a strategy.

One potential reason is the utility of pain for commanding our attention. Who, after all, can ignore the summons of excruciating pain? It may also have something to do with culture. In America, for example, physical symptoms are generally viewed as more acceptable and legitimate than those associated with mental illness. This sometimes results in people simply living with psychological issues because they feel too embarrassed or ashamed to seek help. In contrast, we rarely hesitate to seek care for a problem involving pain. In fact, it is not uncommon for us to openly share such experiences with whoever is willing to listen.

Regardless of the bodymind's motivation for generating an episode of pain, we are not left without options for recourse. The poignant nature of pain is useful in that it forces us to consider new ways of thinking and behaving. This can facilitate a restoration of balance and reduction of pain.

CHAPTER

4

WHAT ARE YOU THINKING?

"Transformation requires a willingness to challenge your basic beliefs."

—Peter Levine

"A man becomes what he thinks about most the time."

—Ralph Waldo Emerson

In earlier chapters, we learned that pain involves both the mind and body, making it a bodymind phenomenon. In this chapter, we will investigate a variety of ways in which the mind, in particular, can influence pain.

The Mind & Health

Self-healing involves the ability of the bodymind to detect imbalance and make the changes required to eliminate it. More generally, self-healing may be viewed as a form of adaptation. For example, if muscles are overworked, as from a vigorous athletic endeavor, they may become depleted and sore because of their inability to fully cope with the demands of the activity. Fortunately, they will not remain in a weakened state, but will recover in such a way that they become stronger and more capable of dealing with future challenges.

Like sore muscles, most everyday injuries will completely heal within a few days to a few weeks, depending on the severity. More serious problems, such as fractures or serious trauma, will obviously take longer. Though some illnesses remain difficult to overcome, for the vast majority, the bodymind appears fully competent to heal itself.

Despite our remarkable capacity for self-healing, we humans, in a way unlike other animals, have the ability to interfere with this process.[1] As a result, "the human being is one of the few members of the animal kingdom that doesn't live 10 to 12 times the age of puberty."[2] As philosopher Friedrich Nietzsche put it, "Man is more sick, uncertain, changeable, and indeterminate than any other animal, there is no doubt of that—he is the sick animal."

This human propensity for illness is echoed by philosopher Ken Wilber. In his book, *Integral Psychology*, Wilber points out that evolution not only makes way for higher levels of consciousness, but also generates more avenues for pathology. As others throughout history have observed, our expanded consciousness contains the potential to be both our best and worst asset. The unique role of the human mind in illness is tackled in Paul Martin's *The Healing Mind*,[3] as well as the intriguingly titled *Why Zebras Don't Get Ulcers*.[4]

In 1991, researchers at Yale conducted a study involving over 2,800 participants entitled "Health Perceptions and Survival: Do Global Evaluations of Health Status Really Predict Mortality?"

Their results indicated that the *best* predictor of a person's survival over the next 10 years was his or her answer to the following question: *What do you think about your health?* The answer to this simple question entailed greater predictive power than physical symptoms, exams and laboratory tests, and lifestyle choices. For example, although people who smoked were twice as likely to die within the next decade as those who did not, those evaluating their health as poor were *seven* times more likely to die than those rating their health as excellent (with other factors being equal). This study points to the ability of our minds to receive and accurately interpret bodily messages regarding our state of health.

Another study examining this mind-health connection looked at the effect of coping style on the immune system of cancer patients. Individuals classified as "fighters" (i.e., "I will beat this cancer and refuse to give up no matter what.") tended to display a hardy and "fighting" immune system, contributing to higher rates of recovery. Conversely, those reporting depression and hopelessness fared less optimally, exhibiting a less desirable immune profile and poorer outcomes.[5]

The phenomenon of conversion disorder serves as yet another telling example. Conversion disorder may entail what appear to be highly concerning symptoms—paralysis, seizures, deafness, blindness, muteness, even loss of neurological reflexes[6]— despite the absence of any detectable physical disease. It is typically associated with prior trauma and may be triggered in times of duress. Once the stress is alleviated, the symptoms may abate in a relatively short period of time. It is important to realize that the symptoms of conversion disorder are real and that these individuals are not merely feigning disease. Rather, the bodymind, after being subjected to prior trauma, is responding to duress by creating symptoms similar to those typically associated with physical pathology.

Culture and Symptom-Concern

In America, it seems that many people become distressed upon experiencing even a single twinge of pain in the lower back region: "Did I injure my back? Is something out of place?" This tendency has been bolstered by our medical system's practice of treating back pain as a serious disease rather than a condition that often resolves itself.[7]

As articulated in Chapters 1 and 2, culture greatly impacts how we interpret our health. More specifically, it defines what conditions and symptoms are to be considered "abnormal," thereby providing a framework for understanding and interpreting our bodily experiences. Unfortunately, when we overly scrutinize our symptoms in light of such a framework, they can become magnified, which only increases the likelihood that we will view them as abnormal. So it appears that excessive concern with symptoms may actually propagate pain and illness.

This is not to suggest that we should ignore all of our symptoms. As discussed in Chapter 3, the bodymind invokes certain experiences to summon our attention and invoke behavior change. Rather, it is important to understand which symptoms may be cause for concern and those which are likely to be benign. Doing so can be a challenging endeavor though, as much of the medical information that is publicly available may be skewed, profit-seeking, or rooted in tradition rather than sound evidence or reasoning.

Mental Imagery

Imagery has played a key role in remedying a myriad of illnesses throughout human history, and is likely a central factor in what many refer to as "miracles." According to Robert Trestman, imagery has consistently been shown to have a direct influence on healing,[8] and has proven especially efficacious in the treatment of cancer.

Let's start with a quick experiment. Imagine sucking on a freshly sliced lemon. If you took my suggestion, it is likely that you experienced an increase in your salivation (this was true for me each time I edited this section!). Likewise, thinking about or observing another person yawning often provokes a yawn, or at least a desire to do so. Both of these are good examples of the power that mental images have for influencing bodily processes. It is also interesting to note that simply imagining an action, such as moving your arm up and down, elicits the same patterns in your brain as if you were actually performing it.

The content of our mental imagery can be influenced by the diagnosis we receive and its related images (e.g. – "ruptured" disc). Since many of us are ill-informed as to the content of our mental imagery, it can be helpful to utilize techniques such as "guided imagery." By uncovering the sorts of images you hold in your mind, it becomes possible to modify them in a fashion that promotes healing.

Related methods for influencing bodily processes include hypnosis and biofeedback. In one intriguing example, individuals learned to control the activation of a single motor nerve cell with the use of electrodes and auditory feedback.[9] The use of such techniques to direct the body in healing is both intriguing and mystifying. At minimum, they call us to more seriously consider the contents of our minds and their effects on our bodily processes.

The Power of Expectations

Though the mind is capable of making us sick, it can just as readily make us better. For instance, it is not uncommon for people to start feeling better just before they are scheduled to visit their physician. One explanation for this could be that the illness just ran its course. However, many times this fails to tell the complete story. An equally plausible reason is that people expect to improve, and that such expectations begin to be fulfilled even prior to the medical consultation.

Research supports this notion that positive expectations, such as hope and optimism, facilitate healing.[10] In contrast, those who are characteristically pessimistic about recovery often remain sick. A pessimistic or cynical attitude may perpetuate a vicious cycle, in which a negative outlook and poor health reciprocally reinforce each other. For ideas on cultivating a more positive outlook, see Appendix II.

The Self-Fulfilling Prophecy

The proverbial "self-fulfilling prophecy" exists when expectations influence future events. This is powerfully illustrated by the example of Voodoo death. In societies where people believe in the power of a curse, death or severe illness may often follow its pronouncement. This probably occurs because these people so strongly expect that something bad will happen to them that it becomes actualized in their bodies.

There are also innumerable anecdotal reports of people dying on or shortly after their birthdays, anniversaries, or other milestones. Although skeptics may dismiss these as coincidental, it appears that something else may be occurring. These people, whether consciously aware of it or not, appear to be strongly motivated by their circumstances, thereby influencing the course of their bodily processes.

The White Coat Prophecy

What I'm calling the "white coat" prophecy is a form of self-fulfilling prophecy in which a clinician's words or manner influence a patient's recovery. This may include things such as impacting the way a patient responds to a drug or to a given diagnosis. If the clinician's outlook appears positive, the patient is more likely to do well than otherwise. For example, in 1861, Dr. John Gunn wrote:

"A lady informed me that opium administered in any way caused her great restlessness, violent headache, and vomiting. Having of necessity to use it in her case...I prescribed it under a new name... I gave her opium for a length of time without producing the least symptoms of headache or vomiting, but on the contrary, she slept soundly and improved in health. She also spoke in the highest terms of this new remedy."

Unfortunately, white coat prophecies can also perpetuate negative outcomes. I regularly come across patients in my physical therapy practice who seem to have worsened as a result of what they were told at a previous healthcare encounter. This is sometimes referred to as iatrogenic illness (physician-induced) or the nocebo effect (the sinister sibling of the placebo effect). From this, I've deduced that many clinicians are either haphazard or ignorant of the power they possess to influence a patient's condition with their words and manner.

For example, by nonchalantly informing a patient that she has degeneration of her spinal discs (without providing further qualification), she may assume that she has a serious medical problem. This may cause her pain to worsen as a result of heightened fear, negative expectations, and the inception of ominous mental images.

Not too long ago, a good friend of mine informed me that a physician had predicted 30 years ago that she would experience progressive arthritis as a result of a hard fall that she had taken. She indicated how that prophecy had remained imprinted in her mind all these years, but that she had always retained an element of skepticism. Recently, she had an X-ray taken of the area and was informed that there was very little arthritis present. Not surprisingly, the overreaching medical prediction had proven erroneous, but it could have induced more noxious consequences had she taken it to heart and transformed it into a self-fulfilling prophecy.

Because of the potential for a clinician's words and manner to negatively impact your health, you should attempt to think critically about what you are told and independently investigate your health concerns.

The Placebo Effect

Closely related to the prophecies described above is what is commonly known as the placebo effect. The placebo effect involves the activation of the body's natural healing resources through the power of beliefs, expectations, or mental imagery. In other words, if you strongly believe that a treatment will help—snake oil, the laying of hands, medications, etc.—it can be effective, regardless of its "actual" potency.

Perhaps what is most interesting about the placebo effect is its ubiquity; the placebo is no respecter of persons. On average, the placebo effect is thought to facilitate improvement in approximately

30-35% of its recipients, regardless of the condition being treated.[11] This means that, on average, a third of those receiving a placebo (often a sugar pill) will show the same improvement as those receiving the actual drug. From this, it does not appear outlandish to suggest that our bodies are innately equipped to do as much as the combined powers of pharmaceutical research have provided us to date, and more. It is for this reason that some historians believe *"The history of medicine is largely the history of the placebo effect."*[12]

The power of the placebo effect is exemplified by a study examining the   effects of surgery on knee pain.[13] The head researcher, Dr. Bruce Moseley, had observed that his patients usually felt better after surgery, but he was curious to discover which portion of the surgery was most responsible for the improvement.

He divided the subjects into three groups: One would have damaged cartilage removed, another would have the knee flushed to remove potential precipitants of inflammation, while the third group would simply be anesthetized and acquire three standard incisions with no surgical intervention (i.e., placebo treatment). Cutting (no pun intended) to the chase, all groups improved, but none of the treatments were significantly superior. Moseley proceeded to report: "My skill as a surgeon had no benefit on these patients. The entire benefit of surgery for osteoarthritis of the knee was the placebo effect."[14]

The "It's Gonna' Hurt" Prophecy: Fear-Avoidance

We are pattern-seeking creatures. In fact, noticing trends is a skill that has been quite instrumental in our evolutionary success, important for activities such as tracking when and where food is most likely to be found. However, our pattern-seeking tendencies can also deceive us, as what appears to be a real cause-effect pattern may be nothing but an illusion or coincidence. Things such as magic, superstitions, and myths thrive upon the human capacity to wholeheartedly trust whatever patterns we detect.

Detecting and trusting apparent patterns can strongly influence the behavior of a person struggling with pain. For instance, you may come to believe that performing a certain activity, such as vacuuming, causes your back pain to become much worse. This is usually based on at least one instance when you performed the activity and the pain seemed to increase as a result. Pain then becomes associated with the activity, in this case vacuuming, and you conclude that it should therefore be avoided.

What I am describing is commonly referred to as "fear-avoidance," in which an activity is avoided due to anticipated pain.[15] Fear-avoidance has been shown to contribute to the development of chronic back pain and disability.[16] Over time, a person may continue to add more activities to his or her "can't do list" until (s)he feels completely helpless and disabled. Here are some examples of fear-avoidance beliefs:

"When I get too tired, I end up in pain."

"If I'm on my feet for more than ten minutes at a time,
I'm in pain the rest of the day."

"I can't have sex because my back pain will be excruciating
the next day."

"I shouldn't bend over because it might throw my back out."

It is important to realize that fear-avoidance conditioning is often based on inaccurate beliefs about pain, as well as our tendency to embrace patterns that may not be real (or become real as self-fulfilling prophecies).[17] Appendix III provides information for overcoming fear-avoidance, which is a critical component in recovering from chronic pain. To further illustrate the importance of our beliefs and behavior toward pain (remember our CEO acronym), consider the following scenarios:

Scenario #1: Judy

Judy first noticed a twinge in her lower back while bending forward to pick up her keys. Over the course of the day, she noticed the pain becoming more frequent and intense. She'd never experienced back pain before, but she had heard that it could become quite severe and potentially disabling. Thus, she grew more concerned about what might be wrong. Over the next few days, Judy could not help but focus on her back, as she tried to rest and protect it from further harm. When the pain continued, she decided to consult with her physician, who seemed concerned that she might have a ruptured disc and proceeded to order an MRI. Judy continued to focus on her back, worrying that each twinge of pain might be a sign that she was making the problem worse. Therefore, she continued to rest and avoided most movements. After the MRI, the doctor explained that she did not have a herniation, but that she did have some degeneration of her discs. When Judy asked about recovery, the physician indicated that he was uncertain, but would give her some medication to see if it would help. He also advised that she continue to take it easy for a while. Judy continued to favor her back and wondered if the pain would ever go away. Since she wasn't doing what she normally enjoyed, she also began to get depressed. The fear, pain, concern, and frustration continued.

Scenario #2: Kim

Kim began to notice pain in her back while at work. She was surprised at how much it hurt, but was confident that it would abate, just as her other aches and pains had in the past. She also realized that she had been under a lot of stress recently and noticed increased tension in her muscles. Therefore, she figured that the stress and tension could feasibly be contributing to the pain in her low back. Over the next few days, Kim tried to stay active despite her back pain. Though she would take rest breaks, she was determined not to let the pain get her down. She also took some measures to decrease her stress, opting to enjoy an extended weekend. By early the next week, the pain had decreased significantly and all that remained was a toothache-like sensation. After a few more days, the ache had subsided and she experienced no further symptoms.

Strategies for Managing a New Onset of Pain

Judy did not demonstrate helpful beliefs or behavior toward pain, nor did her physician. Like many people, she worried that she might have a serious and debilitating injury. She continued to limit her activity levels, which only added to the problem. Kim, on the other hand, demonstrated excellent management strategies. She did not overly concern herself with the pain and adjusted her lifestyle appropriately. By realizing that other factors, such as stress, were probably involved, she was able to remain confident that the pain would disperse in a way similar to previous tension-related issues. Here are some helpful tips for managing pain effectively like Kim:

1) Understand What Causes Pain: Work to fully comprehend the material in this book and/or related resources.

2) Stay Active: Regardless of the cause of pain, it is okay to take it easy for a couple days. After doing so, however, research supports returning to normal movement and activity levels as soon as possible (with the exceptions of major pathologies or injuries, such as a fracture). As we have seen from Judy's story, continuing to rest can foment additional problems, including frustration, loss of physical function, and depression. Since returning to normal activity will not damage the painful area, it is best to set progressive activity goals and measure your progress in terms of function, rather than focusing on pain levels (see Chapter 5 and Appendix III for more on this).

3) Remain Positive: Recovering from an episode of pain may not always involve smooth and consistent improvement. Initially, you may even encounter more bad days than good. Regardless, it helps to attempt to maintain a positive outlook, as the body responds best to hope and optimism. By expecting the best, you will maximize your healing resources. More ideas for cultivating a positive outlook are described in Appendix II.

4) Change the Way You Talk about Pain: If you are going to change the way you think and behave toward pain, you should also change the way you talk about it. Rather than describing it as a permanent medical condition, talk in terms of your current experience. For example, instead of saying "I have a bad back" you might say "I feel sore and tense today." Your words tend to reinforce the way you think as well as how others treat you, both of which influence your bodily processes. So take time to re-evaluate how you go about describing your experience.

Concluding Thoughts: The Mind in Healing

In my estimation, the notion that the mind can heal is no longer a significant subject of debate. Based on the content provided in this chapter, it should now be clear that what goes on in our minds—beliefs, expectations, mental imagery, the direction of our attention, etc.—is critical to what transpires in our bodies. This should come as no surprise, considering the unified nature of our bodyminds. In fact, changing our minds may be one of the most efficient ways for transforming our bodily experiences, including pain. This is exemplified in the pioneering efforts of John Sarno, Bernie Siegel, Norman Cousins, Herbert Benson, and others (see Sources).

One important phenomenon to consider in light of the mind is that of ceremonial healings. In my view, it may not be necessary to invoke any supernatural forces when attempting to understand such occurrences. Rather, these can be viewed as examples of the vast potential of our bodyminds—typically left untapped—to self-correct. A critical component in the process of a healing event is a fervent belief in the healer and treatment, as well as the expectation of a positive outcome. Whether the healing occurs in a public ceremony or through personal prayer, a deep faith or belief is commonly present.

Healing belief involves a state of bodymind openness. This openness allows for physiological responses which are favorable for restoring balance.[18] At times, this may involve the discharge of accumulated energy and tensions that are contributing to the pain or illness.[19] It also seems appropriate to acknowledge the directive influence of our thoughts and mental imagery on the timing of our bodily affairs, whether this involves instantaneous healing, or dying on a date that holds special significance.

Despite the striking potentials of the human mind, it is not entirely clear how or why it plays such a powerful role in healing. Moreover, since mental phenomena are intangible by definition, changing them can sometimes seem difficult. Based on what we've learned in this chapter, however, it can be well worth the effort. It is for this reason that the first letter of our "CEO" acronym exhorts: Change your thoughts and behavior toward pain.

5

RE-THINKING THE BODY

"Beginning in early childhood and throughout life, each of us makes decisions affecting our health. They are made, for the most part, without regard to, or contact with, the health care system. Yet their cumulative impact has a greater effect on the length and quality of life than all the efforts of medical care combined."—1979 Surgeon General Report

As we have been discussing, our goal is to explore an expanded view of pain, as the predominant cultural emphasis on "body as machine" fails to convey the whole story. This does not mean, however, that we should throw out the body out with the bath water. Rather, it is necessary to distinguish what is true about the role of the body in pain from what is merely myth or hearsay. For instance, in Chapter 2, we learned that bodily abnormalities, such as flattened spinal disks, are generally inconsequential with respect to pain.

In this chapter, we will touch on a variety of bodily factors, such as movement and muscle tension, which are germane to our task. We will also discuss some common misconceptions involving the body and pain.

Tension & Pain

Tension, with respect to muscles, indicates the degree to which they are stretched or taut. Tension can also refer to a general bodily state or experience (e.g. - "I feel tense."). Though we sometimes attempt to differentiate psychological tension and muscle tension, they are actually inseparable. If you report feeling tense, what you are describing is an alteration in your body's physiology—specifically, an increase in muscle tone. Tension, like pain and emotions, should therefore be understood as a bodymind phenomenon. It may be for this reason that "stress" is now frequently used to refer to psychological and emotional unease, while "tension" usually retains a bodily connotation.

We are all aware, to varying degrees, of factors that contribute to our daily tensions. Stress from work, relationships, and finances are among the most prevalent. We also carry tensions of which we are unaware, housed in the realms of the subconscious (see Chapter 7).

Tension is not only felt internally, but is also manifested outwardly in our postures, body shape, and demeanor. The contributors to the anthology, *Body, Breath, and Consciousness,* suggest that character development and structure are intricately related to the muscular system. If trauma or other developmental problems affect a muscle group at a critical period, the muscle may acquire an abnormal tone and hamper the subsequent development of associated character traits.

For example, someone with a history of hypotonic (i.e., weakened) extensor muscles in the spine, perhaps manifesting in a slumped posture, is disposed to exhibit signs of depression and lowered self-esteem. The fact that we might call him or her "spineless" probably indicates an intuitive awareness of this mind-body interaction. Other personality descriptors such as uptight, nervous, rigid, unbending, spineless, firm-handed, soft-hearted, and stiff-necked are often not far removed from the bodily characteristics of those they describe.[1] As a result of this instantiation of personality in the body, we tend to assess people very quickly through an unconscious reading of their body language and appearance, supporting the notions of "instant chemistry" and "gut feelings."[2]

Two regional storehouses for tension are the neck & shoulders and the lower back & buttocks. This, in part, helps to account for the high rates of back and neck pain reported in our society. Many people have also come to realize that tension in the back or neck can contribute to symptoms in the limbs. Diagnoses such as tendonitis of the elbow, carpal tunnel syndrome, or various forms of hip and knee pain are not uncommonly related to tension being housed upstream in the back or neck (see Appendix IV). Thus, recognizing sources of tension, even if subtle, can be important when addressing pain.[3]

Related to this discussion is a type of bodywork called "Rolfing," which is often reported to be quite painful. Rolfing practitioners believe that their aggressive massage techniques do not *produce* pain, but merely uncover sources of painful tension in the body. In fact, if the tension is effectively released with a Rolfing treatment, the pain and tenderness is no longer experienced, even when significant pressure is applied.

As a result of my investigations into Rolfing, I became interested to discover where I might be tender to touch and if I may not be unknowingly holding tension in those areas. With exploration, I discovered several areas of tenderness in my abdominal wall. I proceeded to wonder if holding tension in these muscles was related to my tendency toward limiting full expansion of my diaphragm while breathing. Though it is difficult to know such things with certainty, the connection between pain, tenderness, and tension is supported in both theory and practical experience.

Managing Tension

It is probably safe to say that no one participating in modern society can completely eliminate daily tensions. We might more realistically speak of managing or reducing tension. If you recall the concept of bodymind threshold introduced in Chapter 3, it may only take a small reduction in your tension (or other imbalances) to significantly modify your pain experience. Since addressing tension can alleviate pain, I offer the following strategies for doing so:

1) Increase your awareness of your body and your tension: Though most of us are aware of at least one region of the body where we hold tension, it can be useful to map out your tension more thoroughly. The more areas of tension that you can uncover, the better off you will be. By increasing your ability to sense your tension, you can more readily learn to consciously relax the area.

There are many routes to increasing your awareness. Movement is one such route, which will be discussed below. Meditation and other bodymind practices can also be quite effective (see Chapter 6 & Appendix I). One frequently overlooked awareness-enhancer is touch, such as massage and other forms of bodywork. Though touch is commonly used to address muscle tension, its benefits are not limited to increased circulation and other physiological changes. Touch also serves to heighten awareness of bodily sensations and feelings. In this sense, touch is like a mirror into the forgotten territories of your body, serving to reengage your awareness of how they feel and function. Massage can reinvigorate bodily regions that were previously experienced as numb and lifeless. In some cases, touch may precipitate a powerful emotional release, which serves to demonstrate its power to increase awareness, even of distant emotional memories.

Maintaining an ongoing awareness of your bodymind and your environment is sometimes referred to as "mindfulness"—the diametric opposite of living on autopilot. Mindfulness in this sense involves paying attention to the state of your bodymind throughout the day, including the sensations, impulses, thoughts, and feelings you experience. As your mindfulness increases, you will become more aware of messages from your body asking you to move a certain way, apply touch, change positions, and so on. When such messages are blocked or go unnoticed, your body has no choice but to remain tense and out of touch with your awareness.

2) Identify contributors to your tension and learn to manage it on the fly: Once you become more in-tune with your tension, you will be better prepared to identify why and what you are tensing. Factors contributing to tension can generally be grouped into two categories: outer and inner. Outer sources of tension are typically easy to identify: bosses, in-laws, traffic jams, telemarketers, and the like. Despite the fact that these are not always controllable, you do have a choice in how you respond to such stressors. Inner contributors to tension may include your thoughts, worries, stress and anxiety levels, as well as any tensing patterns that you are maintaining unknowingly. Mindfulness of these factors will increase your ability to address your tension in its infancy before it snowballs and crosses the pain threshold.

3) Set aside time to address accumulated tension: Since it is sometimes difficult to completely diffuse tension as it occurs, it helps to set aside time specifically for relaxing and unwinding. Though there is no right or wrong way to reduce your tension, some methods will probably be more effective for you than others. What is most important is discovering something that you enjoy doing.

My sessions usually consist of a combination of mindful movements, relaxing in different postures, and seated or lying relaxation. My preferred time is around dusk (although many people prefer early mornings). I spend anywhere from ten minutes to ninety minutes, depending on how I feel and how much time is available. Though I prefer to be alone during these sessions, you may enjoy participating with others, such as taking a yoga class or savoring a massage from your mate. Afterward, I typically feel lighter, more relaxed, and balanced—a perfect prelude to sleep.

Regardless of your particular routine, it should be a time of simply enjoying "you" from the inside, a celebration of the sensations and experiences of your bodymind. As you do so more regularly, you will notice a decrease in your regularly felt levels of tension, as well as a heightened sense of well-being.

Movement is Fundamental

Movement is the foundation of life and the universe; nothing is ever entirely static. Rather, all things are dynamically interacting with each other, a vast cosmic dance party. Our bodies are no different.

Our physiology depends on movement, an economy of mingling molecules. Considering the macro level, movement allows us to attain food and shelter, defend ourselves, reproduce, engage in relationships, and negotiate our environments. It also provides a means for self-expression, for communicating our inner needs and longings to the world around us.

Since movement is fundamental to our livelihood, it should come as no surprise that hindered or restricted movement can be detrimental and painful. Unfortunately, it has become commonplace for us to move with diminished frequency, spontaneity, and sophistication as we age.

As early as grade school, we are told that certain movements or postures are unacceptable: "Sit up straight. Stop fidgeting. Sit still." Restriction of movement frequently continues into adulthood, at which time we begin to believe that certain types of movements are no longer feasible. Surely you've heard people remark "I'm getting too old for that," or "I can't do that anymore." Though there may be some truth to these statements for particular individuals, such limitations appear to result more from habitual choices than any form of biological determinism.

Without being too idealistic, the fact is that we are selling ourselves short when we give up participating in complex and challenging movements. Highly-skilled movements *can* be maintained throughout life, assuming that you are willing to invest some time and attention. Even in cases where a person has significantly impaired movement, much of the original capacity can be restored because of the inherent adaptability of the bodymind.

Movement & Pain

In addition to restrictions imposed by "sitting still" and the supposed limitations of old age, conventional wisdom often advises us to stop moving following an onset of pain or injury. In contrast to this practice, those who begin to move shortly after injury display faster recovery times.[4] Similarly, people who continue to perform their jobs recover more effectively and are less likely to file for disability than those who take extended time off.[5]

Such findings have influenced the recommended clinical guidelines for managing low back pain in both the U.S. and U.K., which now advocate early return to activity.[6] Though there are exceptions, soft tissue injuries (e.g. – sprains, strains, etc.) generally respond best to progressive movement and activity.[7] The use of medication and heat/cold applications can be helpful for reducing pain and making movement more palatable following an injury.

As stated above, our bodies are highly adaptable, allowing even the most engrained movement deficiencies to be overcome, as well as related pain. As a practicing physical therapist, I regularly observe the importance of movement with respect to healing. I have noticed that people who choose to minimize their movement or activity level (opting instead to immobilize the painful area) often experience the most pain and dysfunction. After I help them to move more freely and return to their usual activities, they typically report a significant reduction in pain.

From these observations, I've come to believe that when we fail to move, the bodymind will continue to detect and signal an imbalance, regardless of the state of tissue healing. This perceived imbalance, along with its concomitant discomfort, resolves once normal movement and activities are resumed.

Although the therapeutic benefits of movement are evident with most tissue injuries, the common ankle sprain is perhaps the most instructive example. Generally, in order to recover from a mild or moderate ankle sprain, a person should initiate walking within a few days of the injury. Granted, there will be some pain involved, but walking will slowly become easier and less painful. Within a week or two, the ankle usually feels nearly normal again.

We can derive similar wisdom from observing animals who, following an injury, may limp for only a few hours/days (or not at all) before they are up and running again. The moral of the story is that it is often beneficial to move, even in the presence of some pain, in order to recover. If you try to wait until the pain is gone before you start moving, you may be waiting a long time.

Some people wonder if healing will be impeded if the injured area continues to be moved. In response to this reasonable question, think about what happens after scraping a knuckle. You do not stop bending the finger, worrying that it will never heal, but intuitively know that it will heal even with active use. The same principle applies to other areas of the body, which is why physical therapists (at least this one) do not hesitate to prescribe progressive movement following most injuries. Among other things, movement ensures that the injured area retains its ability to move fluidly as it heals.

Despite the importance of restoring normal movement following injury, it is usually wise to proceed gradually. This can be done intuitively, such as alternating sensible activity with the felt need for rest. Or, for those exhibiting chronic pain and fear-avoidance, you may wish to construct a more formal activity plan. This might involve setting progressive activity goals and working toward accomplishing them, even in the presence of pain (see Appendix III for more on this).

I especially encourage you to move spontaneously, creatively, and mindfully. So much of our daily movement and posturing tends to be culturally-dictated, to the extent that we have forgotten how to express ourselves through bodily movement. As I discuss in Chapter 7, self-expression is critical to good health, and movement is one of the most effective ways of doing so. So even if you don't feel comfortable moving freely in the presence of others (which seems to be true for most people), try to find a time and place where you can move in an open, unfettered fashion.

Nature & Nurture

These days, it is difficult to travel far without encountering discussions of "nature and nurture." Such discussions often evoke questions such as these: Are we smart because of our genes or because of our educational opportunities? Are health problems heritable or are they linked to diet or other lifestyle factors? And so on.

In our society, functioning largely under the body-machine story, it seems that genes receive a disproportionate amount of the credit. The problems with this bias are highlighted in Dr. Bruce Lipton's *The Biology of Belief*, which describes how contextual factors are instrumental in determining how genes are expressed. Lipton advocates for a more recent field of biology called epigenetics, which examines biological control mechanisms that function relatively independently of genes.

The fact that our health is contingent on a variety of conditional factors can entail both positive and negative consequences. For example, a child whose prenatal and postpartum environments are highly stressful will develop a physiology that is hypersensitive and hyper-reactive to stress. This physiological molding can be difficult to overcome as an adult, predisposing the individual to chronic activation of the stress response and related illnesses. Though at first this may sound undesirable and perhaps even unfair, this is nature's way of our ensuring survival under threatening conditions. Possessing a highly sensitive stress response allows a person to quickly react to imminent threats. In contrast, a calmer individual under similar circumstances may fail to aptly respond to such threats and thereby encounter troublesome consequences.

Because of the interdependent and nuanced relationship between nature and nurture, it is often difficult to clearly identify which is most responsible for an illness. For instance, a woman may report experiencing the same type of back troubles as her mother, attributing the problem solely to genetics. However, by doing so, she may effectively overlook other important factors, such as those described in this book, which could be contributing to her pain. In reality, it may be her mother's beliefs and behaviors she inherited— not her mother's back—which are perpetuating her pain experience.

As another example, women, on average, are more susceptible than men to many types of chronic illnesses, such as chronic pain, depression, and various autoimmune disorders. However, we should again exercise caution in attributing these disparities solely to biology. From a cultural standpoint, it is not difficult to see why women may be more prone to such illnesses, as they are often burdened with more extensive responsibilities than men. In many cases, women function not only as full-time mothers, but work outside of the home under less than ideal conditions. Furthermore, the abuse of females, in both childhood and adulthood, far exceeds that of males, predisposing them to ill health. So even when we suspect that we are identifying genetic or physiological differences, we may become more ambivalent upon deeper investigation.

Going Deeper with Diagnosis

In our medical culture, the body-machine mindset tends to dominate when it comes to clinical diagnosis—focusing on germs, genes, and structural abnormalities.   As commonly practiced, this approach appears to preclude deeper reasoning regarding potentially more foundational causes of pain or disease.

For example, if you exhibit elevated blood pressure over successive visits to your physician, you may be diagnosed with hypertension, or high blood pressure. Unfortunately, this diagnosis serves merely as a descriptor, with no reference to any deeper cause. In other words, it fails to address what is causing your blood vessels to constrict or other physiological changes contributing to the elevated measurement.

The body-machine story might suggest that hypertension is related to age or genetics, which does not tell the whole story. After all, it is not highly uncommon for a person recently diagnosed with high blood pressure to have had normal measurements just a year or two ago.   So it seems reasonable to wonder: Why the sudden change? Is such a change permanent? Unfortunately, the body is commonly assumed to be "once bad, forever bad."

But what about deeper causes? As described throughout this book, there are multiple factors that may contribute to pain.   To return to our hypothetical example, high blood pressure may be related to excess body weight, which may in turn be linked with excessive or unhealthy eating.   Poor dietary choices may be a response to depression, loneliness, and/or relational difficulties, any of which may be related to a diminished sense of life purpose or meaning, inadequate social skills, a recent tragedy, or other life troubles. Beyond the contributions of diet to high blood pressure, psychosocial factors alone can precipitate an elevation of blood pressure, as chronic stress may result in the constriction of vascular smooth muscle; thus the term "hyper-*tension*."

So it is this type of probing—done independently or in consultation with a physician, spouse, mental health professional, close friend, etc.—which may be most beneficial, since it attempts to identify the most foundational sources of the problem. We need to ask "why?": Why is my blood pressure high? Why am I stressed-out? And so on.

The Role of Chemistry in Pain

Poor general health is another factor that increases our susceptibility to pain, as alterations in body chemistry may provide a fertile ground for the germination of disease processes. For instance, obesity or diabetes can engender a cascade of changes in chemical processes throughout the body that increase the likelihood of other problems. The chemical effects of inflammation are especially poignant and worthy of our attention.

Though often viewed negatively by clinicians, inflammation does serve a beneficial purpose. Following an injury, the immune system responds with inflammatory chemicals to help repair tissue damage. Inflammation that targets a specific site of injury is known as local inflammation. During this process, inflammatory mediators may sensitize the area, making subsequent movement or pressure uncomfortable. This functions to temporarily protect the area from further injury while the healing process is initiated.

Another type of inflammation is known as low-grade, systemic inflammation. In contrast to local inflammation, systemic inflammation involves the presence of inflammatory chemicals throughout the body. These chemicals have been shown to affect the walls of blood vessels and are correlated with cardiovascular disease, as well as a number of other illnesses such as chronic pain, cancer, obesity, diabetes, digestive disorders, and Alzheimer's disease.[8] A strong potential contributor to systemic inflammation is obesity.[9]

Adipose tissue, commonly known as fat, is highly capable of producing and secreting chemicals involved in inflammation. These chemicals could be responsible, at least in part, for complications associated with obesity, such as diabetes and cardiovascular diseases. In their research review, Nicklas and colleagues highlighted evidence demonstrating weight loss and exercise to significantly mitigate these inflammatory processes as well as their noxious side-effects.[10] Diet may also influence pain, although the extent to which food selection is important (beyond its influence on body fat levels) is not entirely clear.

At this point, I would like to address two common misconceptions related to chemistry and pain. First, the breakdown of cartilage that covers the ends of bones, often mistakenly labeled "arthritis" (which actually refers to joint inflammation), is often implicated as a certain producer of pain. Second, when people experience sharp pain in the neck or lower back, they are often led to believe it is resulting from a "pinched nerve." Here is my rejoinder:

Many people with very little cartilage remaining at their joints report *little or no pain*. I witness this frequently in my physical therapy practice. Even when joints are grinding, crunching, or popping, people often report they are not painful. This is supported by the research I presented in Chapter 2.

With regard to nerve "pinching," our nerves are pinched or stretched—which is to say, compressed or elongated—with every movement we make, and are fully capable of enduring such forces without sustaining injury. So to implicate routine compression (i.e., "pinching") as the primary cause of pain appears rather spurious.[11]

But what causes shooting pains and aching joints? In addition to the contributions of other factors described throughout this book, these phenomena may be related to chemical irritation of nerves, which increases their sensitivity to what are normally painless forces such as compression or stretching. This chemical irritation may be related to inflammation, stress-related chemicals, altered tissue pH, or some combination thereof.[12] In other words, pain is sometimes more of a chemical issue than a mechanical one, since a sensitized nerve may become painful even under normal physical forces.

As a result of the role of chemistry, particularly inflammation, in pain, the use of anti-inflammatory medications may often be beneficial, especially in cases of injury or exacerbated arthritis. By reducing the level of chemical irritants, returning to daily activities becomes more tolerable and recovery is expedited. Anti-inflammatories are more effective when taken on a scheduled basis for a period of time (as opposed to as needed), which allows them to build to a potent level in the body. Ideally though, these medications should be discontinued (or at least diminished) shortly after the pain is reduced to a more palatable level.

Does Repetitive Activity Cause Premature Bodily Breakdown?

Following the logic of the body-machine story, it is commonly suggested that repetitive or intense physical activity contributes premature bodily breakdown and pain. This belief, which I call the "wear and tear" myth, has failed to be substantiated by research. In fact, research seems to support the opposite effect, in that regular physical activity appears to contribute to bodily durability and longevity.

For instance, people who run several miles a week do not display joint degeneration any more frequently or quickly than non-runners.[13] In fact, distance running may actually have a *protective* effect on joint integrity.[14] One study concluded that "older persons who engage in vigorous running and other aerobic activities have lower mortality and disability."[15] The same appears to be true for those who keep their minds active, as regular mental exercise may delay the onset of dementia and other problems. Essentially, the evidence tends to lend greater support to the proverbial "use it or lose it" concept.

In concert with the body-machine story and the "wear and tear" myth is the notion of overuse or "repetitive stress" injury. For example, if a person regularly performs computer work and suddenly begins to experience wrist pain, it is frequently assumed to be a case of carpal tunnel syndrome. Or, if a factory worker complains of elbow pain, it is thought to be "tennis elbow."

I am not disputing the fact that irritated tissues can be painful, nor arguing that repetitive motion is inherently good for our physical or mental health. However, it does appear that diagnoses of overuse have become, well, overused (sorry), almost to the point of becoming the default for anyone who has pain and also happens to perform repetitive or strenuous work. Moreover, the validity of overuse injuries has not been substantiated in research or in legal proceedings, leading some researchers to understand them as primarily sociocultural phenomena.[16]

I reason that if a painful problem is truly related to inflammation, such as a case of tendonitis or muscle strain, then the problem should abate with a few days of rest and attempts to reduce the inflammation. Unfortunately, in many cases, workers fail to improve even when significantly longer rest periods are provided. This discrepancy seems to imply that factors beyond overuse are at play. For example, if you recall from Chapter 2, psychosocial factors, such as job perceptions, may better predict who will develop work-related pain, as well as who will progress to chronic dysfunction and disability.[17]

Before moving on, I wished to clarify that certain behaviors and circumstances do appear to precipitate premature aging and bodily breakdown. Things such as the perception and actuality of a "hard life" (i.e., enduring poverty, abusive relationships, and other harsh circumstances), nutritional deficits, morbid obesity, etc., can all contribute to untimely and sometimes rapid deterioration of health.

It is important to recognize, however, that stress depends largely on the perceptions of the beholder, as circumstances that may overwhelm or frighten one person may be viewed as a challenge to be transcended by another. Our outlook and coping capacities account for much of the variance in regard to how our bodies will be affected. If you view your life as taxing and difficult, your body will tend to register it that way; if you see it as challenging and enjoyable, it is likely to respond more favorably.

A Word on Posture

While in training as a physical therapist, I was taught that "poor posture" contributes to a variety of painful problems. This assertion is not surprising, considering that the physical therapy profession approaches pain primarily from the body-machine perspective (after all, it is *physical* therapy). Since my days in graduate school, my position on posture (pardon the pun) has deviated, to a certain extent, from the conventional wisdom. There are a few reasons I struggle with situating posture high on the priority list with respect to managing pain.

First, what "ideal posture" entails is debatable. I agree with Feldenkrais[18] that what is critical is possessing effective options for movement. In this sense, ideal posture is not attaining and holding a certain position, but having the freedom to move should one feel the need to do so. You would be hard-pressed to find a person who actually enjoys sitting in any single position for an extended period of time, regardless of the posture. It seems then that the ability to move freely and effectively should comprise a greater share of our attention.

Next, biomechanical posturing rarely appears to be a determinative factor in most painful conditions. If this were the case, it seems that 98% of the population would be in pain, since few of us are highly conscientious in this regard. This has been substantiated in my clinical experience, in that postural "abnormalities," such as flat feet, are rarely altered significantly through treatment, yet the pain often abates just as readily. So it appears rather untenable to argue for posture as the primary cause of such problems.

The last thing I wished to mention is the potential for postural nitpicking to create paranoia or fear-avoidance behavior. In other words, if we are told that pain is caused by our posturing, we will worry that any deviation from perfection may foment pain. Rather than helping the problem, then, emphasizing posture may actually make a painful condition worse, not to mention its negative effects on our enjoyment of life in general. In this light, it is unfortunate that most "back safety" programs continue to do exactly that, leading people to believe that their backs and bodies are fragile and incapable of performing any significant amount of physical work unless a rigidly prescribed posture can be maintained.

With that said, I do believe that there are reasons we should take posture into consideration. First, posture influences our overall sense of well-being. Take a minute and exaggerate a slump down into your chair. Most likely, if assumed long enough, you will begin to feel rather lifeless. In a slouched or slumped position, your breathing is restricted and internal organs compressed. Now, sit or stand tall with head up and shoulders back. Notice the increased freedom of your breath and subsequent increase in alertness and vitality. The influence of our posturing on how we feel is yet another aspect of the mind-body connection.

Over time, our postural tendencies may also reshape our bodies. Posture reflects more than genetics, as our bodies are constantly adapting and reforming themselves. You can therefore understand your current bodily form as a partial reflection of your previous life experiences, posturing, and circumstances.[19] For instance, a person with chronic depression will often present with a slumped spine and rounded shoulders, suggesting a burdened or collapsing inner world.[20] Because of the integrated nature of the bodymind, changing your posture can improve your both your psychological and physiological well-being..

Overall, it appears that maintaining a relaxed, upright posture can be beneficial for mind, body, and emotions. The great yogis (notorious for their mind-body unity) have consistently emphasized the role of posture as part of an effective spiritual discipline. An upright posture also appears desirable from a physical standpoint, in that it may help to reduce postural deformities related to bone conditions such as osteoporosis, while providing the opportunity for full and unfettered breathing. Posture is important then, but for different reasons than normally supposed.

Concluding Thoughts

Our bodies are not static and fragile entities disposed to break when moved the wrong way. In fact, we are comprised mostly of fluid, which nicely illustrates our propensity for ongoing adaptation and flexibility, including our capacity for self-healing. It is time for us to move beyond the body as machine-concept and begin re-thinking our stories about the body.

6

STRESS, PERSONALITY, & RELATIONSHIPS

Dr. George Valliant followed two hundred Harvard graduates for 30 years. Comparing the happiest to the unhappiest he reported: "Of the 59 men with the best mental health...only two became chronically ill or died by the age of 53. Of the 48 men with the worst mental health...18 became chronically ill or died."—Bernie Siegel

All entities are, to varying extents, products of their environments. We like to picture ourselves as the exception, as creatures of inexorable free will, dictating our own destinies. Though we display greater freedom than other forms of life, it seems important to acknowledge that our thoughts and behaviors are not all our own. We saw in the first chapter how predominant cultural stories often undergird our personal stories and can thereby influence our state of health and well-being.

In addition to the body-machine story, "The American Dream" represents a central narrative in our culture. This story, in my conception, confuses the pursuit of happiness with the acquisition of material gain. As a result, Americans work longer hours with far fewer vacation days than most Europeans, leaving less time for relationships and recreational endeavors. This can be quite burdensome and stressful for many people, particularly those without the financial means, opportunities, or abilities necessary to satisfy such ideals. The single-mother working for minimum wage, while at the same time attempting to raise children, is one of innumerable examples.

Since such distress does not go unnoticed by the bodymind, it is not surprising that those who are socioeconomically poor are more than twice as likely to report their health as poor.[1] Distress may be especially prevalent in those who have emigrated from other cultures, as difficulty understanding and communicating within a new culture may exacerbate everyday concerns and frustrations.

These difficulties spill over into healthcare as well, since each culture carries a different way of understanding—a different story—about the causes and remedies of illness. Though human biology may be fairly consistent across cultures, diversity in how health and illness are interpreted can introduce further challenges to the provision of effective healthcare.[2]

Stress & Pain

In order to survive, we must possess ways of protecting ourselves against potential threat or danger. Under such circumstances, we utilize what is commonly called "fight-or-flight," a physiological state which quickly initiates when a threat is perceived. More recently, we have come to know this heightened state of reactivity as "stress." We all realize that stress is not restricted to physical threats, but has also become a normative part of everyday modern life.

Closely related to stress are tension and anxiety. These arise, at least in part, when we are confronted with thorny decisions. When we teeter between two equally viable options, we often worry about the repercussions of either choice. This internal tug-of-war generates muscle tension which may accumulate until the issue is put to rest. If you're like me, during times of stress you can feel this tension building in different areas of your body. The muscles of the head, neck, jaw, and back are commonly involved.

We also experience stress when we perceive our circumstances to be out of our control. This may include concerns such as losing a job, not knowing what will be on a final examination, feeling like there is too much to be done in a limited period of time, wondering about the outcomes of a serious illness, etc. What underlies the stress of these situations is fear. We are afraid of failure, afraid of pain, afraid of death, afraid of the unknown. So ultimately, stress is rooted in our fears and concerns about the future.

Stress is often related to external circumstances, like those listed below, which we encounter throughout our lives. It can also be largely internal, related to our physiological conditioning and personality traits. With regard to personality, the extremes of perfectionism and dysfunctional altruism are particularly salient contributors to stress. Most people are familiar with perfectionism, which we will discuss below. Dysfunctional altruism describes a tendency to try to please everyone while ignoring your own needs.

Both perfectionism and dysfunctional altruism can engender stress and negative emotions, while contributing to a variety of painful conditions.[3]

In Chapter 3, we looked at the question of why people may suddenly experience intense bouts of pain, introducing the concept of threshold as a means of understanding such experiences. Here, I would like to suggest that, in many of cases, stress can be a primary factor in crossing the pain threshold. In fact, you may have already noted this connection, perhaps observing how your pain worsens under stress.

This pain-stress connection is not difficult to understand once we realize that stress is not only psychological, but is also a powerful physical phenomenon, involving a cascade of physiological changes and a heightening of muscle tension (see Appendix VI). These changes serve not only to prepare us for flight-or-fight, but are poignant indicators of imbalance in the bodymind. If the stress is chronic, lasting several weeks or longer, the bodymind has few choices but to generate pain or illness, as it will use whatever means necessary to stimulate a change in behavior toward the restoration of balance.[4]

So please take a minute to think about circumstances preceding a time in your life when you experienced a sudden onset of pain or illness. Be sure to think as far back as weeks or even months prior to the onset of the problem. With some examination, you may recall that you were, stressed, worried, angry, depressed, experiencing relational difficulties, sleep-deprived, etc. Regardless of the stressor, your immune system can become significantly depressed under sustained periods of stress. Research indicates that the following circumstances are often perceived as highly stressful and can thereby play a central role in crossing the pain threshold:

- Death of a friend or loved one
- Marriage, separation, or divorce
- Losing/changing jobs, unemployment, or retirement
- Trauma, including emotional trauma
- Moving, buying a home, or refinancing
- Child leaving home
- Relational difficulties
- Beginning or ending school
- Pregnancy
- Vacations and holidays
- Other major life changes
- Other circumstances involving a perceived loss

Stress Management Strategies

Though I believe that humans can adapt to nearly any circumstance, sometimes it is more reasonable to simply avoid or remove the source of potential stress. For instance, if you grew up in a rural area and your urban job seems like a nightmare, you may benefit from re-examining your priorities and transitioning to more familiar surroundings. If this option appears less prudent, it becomes necessary to learn to how to more effectively manage your response to various stressors. Though it is difficult to completely eliminate stressful circumstances, improving your ability to manage stress is certainly feasible and well worth the effort. Here are some suggestions:

1) Assume control and responsibility for your stress: It is easy to believe that stress is something that just happens to us and is outside the realm of our control. Under this belief, we may feel a sense of helplessness or victimization. Upon closer examination, however, it is clear that we do have a say in how we respond to stress. This is a first and critical step in stress management: acknowledge that you can exercise control over your stress. As Howard Brody put it, "Start to see yourself as a person who is taking charge and less as a person to whom unhealthy things just happen."[5]

2) Increase your bodymind awareness: Though at times it can seem difficult to control your stress response, with practice, anyone can improve. In order to do so, it is useful to develop an awareness of what triggers your stress response and how it manifests in your body. There is accumulating evidence supporting the efficacy of bodymind awareness activities for reducing stress and pain, while increasing overall health and well-being.[6] One study demonstrated a 79% reduction in pain and 80% improvement in self-rated ability to handle stress with meditation.[7]

A good place to begin this process is developing an awareness of your breathing. Yoga, meditation, martial arts, dance, relaxation training, and other activities can also serve to enhance your bodymind awareness. There are innumerable books available describing a variety of techniques, although they are not required. What is required is the intent to increase your awareness and the discipline to practice doing so. There is no right or wrong way, so experiment to see what works for you. It is actually through experimentation—trial and error—that we often learn most effectively. To aid you in beginning this process, I have included some introductory activities in Appendix I.

If you tend to be more analytically-minded, you may also wish to compile a list of all of your fears and concerns. Divide the list into two columns, listing in one the things that you can/will change and in the other those which you cannot. Such a list can serve as a reminder of the futility of worrying about things over which you possess little control.

3) Learn to Breathe Fully: How we breathe significantly influences our levels of tension, stress, and anxiety. When we maintain an awareness of how we are breathing, we are more likely to be aware of other bodymind processes, such as tension, and are better equipped to maintain a relaxed and healthy way of being. In this section, I will describe how to improve the quality of your breathing, but first, I wished to comment more on the origins of our breathing inadequacies.

For the first several years of our lives, most of us are breathing as nature intended, by fully engaging our diaphragm muscle. If you get a chance, pause to observe how a toddler or young child breathes. What is usually apparent is that the majority of the inspiratory expansion and movement occurs in the abdominal region as a result of diaphragm movement.

In contrast, many adults have come to restrict their abdominal expansion and breathe primarily with the chest muscles. One potential reason for this is our society's focus on the washboard abdomen, causing many of us, knowingly or not, to begin holding in our bellies. This act of "holding it in" may also arise out of the belief that abdominal expansion can cause the overlaying muscles to become stretched and loose.

Also significant to our altered breathing patterns are stress and anxiety. When we are stressed or anxious, inhibited breathing can serve to restrain the expression of those emotional states. Thus, someone who is anxious or fearful will tend to breathe more rapidly, shallowly, and partially. If the stress or anxiety becomes chronic, this pattern of breathing may become habitually engrained. A sensible starting point for undoing these dysfunctional patterns is learning to breathe with your diaphragm.

As the name suggests, diaphragmatic breathing involves using the diaphragm to draw air into the lungs. The diaphragm is a broad muscle at the bottom of the ribcage whose primary function is respiration. Diaphragmatic breathing uses less energy than other means, as it effectively draws air deep into the lungs without needing to lift the weight of the ribcage.

To ensure that you are breathing with your diaphragm, lightly place your hand on your abdomen (lying on your back is a good position to learn this) and allow your belly to expand outward with each inhalation (it may initially feel like you are purposely pushing your belly outward) and back inward on exhalation. As you progress in your learning, you may notice that you are breathing less frequently, as greater quantities of oxygen penetrate more deeply into the lungs. You may also experience a sense of relaxation throughout your body, as it is rewards you for the quality of your breathing. Try not to get discouraged. It may take a couple weeks (assuming you're practicing regularly!) before it feels more natural. Remember, you may be challenging nearly a lifetime of engrained patterns, so don't be too hard on yourself.

The benefits of attending to your breathing are magnificent. First, it induces bodily relaxation, serving to lessen stress and anxiety. As with meditation, by focusing on your breathing, you can "breathe away" many of your stress-provoking thoughts. Deeper breathing also massages the vital organs and the lumbar spine, helping to maintain their suppleness and healthy functioning.

4) Get adequate sleep: Inadequate quality or quantity of sleep can exacerbate stress and other bodymind imbalances. Research shows that those who are sleep-deprived often consume more calories, and experience the following: cravings for unhealthy foods,[8] difficulty concentrating, mood swings, stress, anxiety, and other problems.[9] Sleep deprivation has also been shown to increase inflammatory chemicals which can exacerbate pain.[10]

5) Engage in regular physical activity: When contending with stress or anxiety, physical activity can serve as a healthy outlet. In part, the stress relief associated with exercise may be due to the release of the body's natural "feel-good" chemicals called endorphins (these are also released with a good hearty laugh), which regulate mood and facilitate a heightened sense of well-being. Physical activity is associated with a myriad of other health benefits as well, such as lowering body fat (which by itself is important to health) and increasing longevity. Dietary factors, such as caffeine intake, may also play a role in stress, although the extent of their contribution is not entirely clear.

Personality Factors

In all of our interpersonal endeavors, we attempt to understand the minds of others, seeking to identify their motives and dispositions. In doing so, things such as stereotypes and personality types have come to infiltrate our social minds. For instance, the notorious Type-A personality, ostensibly related to heart disease, entails traits such as hurriedness, hostility, aggressiveness, and the desire for control and power. Most likely, you have encountered people exhibiting such an amalgamation of traits.

For a variety of reasons, personality and psychological research can be difficult to accept with a high degree of confidence (humans are just so darn complicated!). Nonetheless, there seems to be adequate evidence, at least in my view, of the negative effects of certain personality factors on health, including pain. These will be described next.

Depression: Depression can be related to several different factors, including stressful life circumstances, disposition, and lack of perceived meaning or purpose in life. Research has implicated depression as a significant factor in the development of many types of pain and illness. This may result from the fact that depression involves a concomitant alteration in our physiology, particularly notable in the immune system. In a similar way, pain and illness may contribute to feeling depressed, which again demonstrates the reciprocal interplay between mind and body.

Anxiety: Mild to moderate levels of anxiety can actually prove beneficial, providing a healthy tension that drives motivation and productivity. However, chronic worry and over-activation of the body's stress response can contribute to pain, excessive tension, and a myriad of bodymind conditions (see Appendix IV).

Feeling Helpless: Research has demonstrated, in both humans and animals, the harmful effects of feeling helpless and without a sense of control over circumstances. In many cases, helplessness may involve inadequate social support and depression. The maladaptive belief that past circumstances dictate the course of one's life may also contribute to perceived helplessness.

Perfectionism: Perfectionism involves standards you set for yourself and for others. If your self-standards are too stringent, you may experience self-blame, lowered self-esteem, and frustration. If your standards for others are too high, you may experience a persistent sense of frustration, anger, and irritation. Though the negative emotions that may accompany perfectionism can contribute to ill health, they may vary greatly among individuals. Those who are able to satisfy their own high standards, for instance, may actually encounter positive health benefits. Therefore, as with most personality factors, it is important to examine how your personality characteristics are working for you, rather than merely assuming them good or bad.

Lack of Self-Expression/Assertiveness: Some people can cope effectively with stressful circumstances without outwardly expressing emotions. Others, who feel the need to express themselves but feel they can or should not, will find themselves at risk for ill health. This inhibition is common in those who exhibit dysfunctional altruism or worry about the ramifications of self-expression.

Chronic Anger/Hostility: This appears to be one of the primary factors contributing to the putative association between the Type-A personality and cardiovascular disease. Anger, like any emotion, can be an appropriate response to certain circumstances. However, when one carries a regularly hostile or frustrated demeanor, it can contribute to chronic activation of the stress response and subsequent health problems.

Extraversion/Introversion: Extraversion describes those who are inclined to be outgoing and gain energy from being around people. Introverts tend to be more reserved and may require significant time alone to recharge. Research has shown that extraverts tend to perceive less pain and use more active coping strategies than those inclined toward introversion.[11] Extraverts also tend to experience more positive emotions and score higher on measures of life satisfaction,[12] while demonstrating decreased levels of physiological reactivity to external stimulation.[13] However, the ostensible health benefits of extraversion are difficult to distinguish from a culture which values extraverted traits. In other words, extraverts may appear healthier because they find it easier to mesh in an increasingly active and social world.

Introverts, on the other hand, may be more prone to certain types of pain and illness because of a perceived incongruence with the extraverted world around them. This is not to say that extraverts are exempt from painful conditions. In fact, research suggests that extraverts exemplify a greater disparity between their physiological states and their subjective experience.[14] Knowingly or not, extraverts may suppress negative emotions and supplant them with positive thinking. So extraverts may be less aware of potentially harmful physiological stress and more disposed to problems related to subconscious emotions (see Chapter 7).

Regardless of whether you are more introverted or extraverted, it is unnecessary and probably futile to attempt to change your personality. With that said, extraverts may benefit from practicing introspection and enhancing their bodily awareness. Introverts may wish to find strategies for improving social competence or create a niche where extraverted traits are not as critical. If appropriate changes are instated, you may enjoy significant improvements in your health, including diminished pain.

Social Support & Intimacy

"Let yourself go, let your emotions come out...and be not afraid of the consequences."—Geertje Brakel, cancer survivor

"The rise in morbidity from social isolation is equal to that of cigarette smoking."—Martha McClintock, University of Chicago

The importance of healthy relationships to both our physical and mental health cannot be over-emphasized. Those with good social support enjoy greater longevity and recover more quickly from illness.[15] One study found that breast cancer patients participating in support group therapy lived twice as long as those who did not participate.[16] This may point to the reason why humans are often regarded as social animals: we depend on the presence of others for engendering a sense of security, identity, health, and well-being.

Dr. Dean Ornish, cardiologist, researcher, and author of the book, *Love and Survival*, has extensively studied the effects of love and relational intimacy on heart disease. He has found that those who learn to express their feelings and experience a deeper sense of intimacy can greatly reduce cardiovascular symptoms. In fact, Dr. Ornish suggests that this is among the most critical factors for improving both the length and quality of his patients' lives. He reports that those who "open their hearts" often do as well (or better) as those undergoing heart surgery. Dr. Ornish recommends that all of his heart patients get involved in support groups where they can learn to better express themselves and listen to others do the same.

Finally, it is important to recognize that good health is not merely an absence of the negative, but an embrace of the positive. Opening our hearts goes far beyond relational love and intimacy, and encompasses things such as gratefulness, forgiveness, faith, hope, and trust. Moreover, we should not limit our conception of relationships to only the interpersonal variety. When we deeply relate or connect to anything—nature, music, animals, a higher power, art, literature, etc.—we can experience an enhanced sense of wholeness and meaning. Generally speaking, it appears that those things that engender a sense of fulfillment and connectedness are also what make us healthy.

7

EXPRESS YOURSELF:
PAIN & EMOTIONS

"Fear, love, and anger are all normal...Whether an emotion is good or bad depends on whether it is appropriate...When a person has two or three conflicting emotions...then he is literally mixed up physiologically and psychologically."—David Fink

"When psychologists speak of the unconscious, it is the body they are talking about." —F.M. Alexander

Whether we realize it or not, we are like walking, breathing databases. Every cell in our bodies has the capacity to store information—to learn—from prior events. This capacity for learning is critical to our survival, as we gather information about our environment and adapt accordingly.

Information that we can readily recall is said to be part of our "conscious" memory. This may include things such as phone numbers, names, faces, etc. Information that is not readily accessible is often said to be "subconscious," suggesting that it is below ("sub") our awareness. Since we all occasionally experience difficulty accessing our memories (i.e., "memory block"), it seems reasonable to assert that much of our memory is stored subconsciously. As a result, accessing a distant memory may require a specific trigger to bring it to consciousness. For example, you have likely experienced various smells or other sensual stimuli that have conjured "forgotten" memories.

Emotions and memories are stored not only in the brain, but in the body. Through her research efforts, Dr. Candace Pert has demonstrated that our emotional framework does not reside exclusively in the brain, but is distributed throughout the entire body. The creation of an emotion depends on the binding of certain molecules, called neuropeptides, to specific cellular receptors. When such binding occurs, there is a shift in the overall state of the bodymind which we have come to call emotion.

An overarching purpose of this emotional network is to inspire appropriate action. The word "emote" is comprised of "e-," meaning "out," and "mote" which connotes movement. Thus, emotions involve a "moving out." This movement-orientated nature of emotions is supported by the fact that emotions are not something we think, but something we feel in the body. Feelings are produced by movements of our muscles and molecules that prompt us to act in a certain way. For instance, sadness often invokes crying, while fear promotes tensing of muscles in preparation for action.

Plastic surgeon Loren Eskenazi, in the intriguing anthology *Consciousness and Healing*, testifies to this muscle-emotion link. In her reflective essay, she describes her observations with a patient who had received a Botox injection in her lips. Following the injection, the patient experienced a temporary paralysis of one of her facial muscles involved with smiling. The woman proceeded to experience powerful emotional memories, including reliving incidents where her parents told her that she needed to smile more often. Obviously, this response was not expected by the patient or physician, but it serves to illustrate the powerful role that even the smallest muscles play in our emotional framework.

Blocked Emotions & Pain

As a result of the integrated nature of body and emotions, it doesn't require a vivid imagination to see how emotions might influence pain or other bodily symptoms. To better understand this relationship, consider an analogy:

Imagine making deposits into bank account without ever making a withdrawal. What would happen to the money? It would continue to accumulate interest and grow into a very large sum. Now, imagine what might happen if emotions and related muscle tension are generated in your body over time, but are never granted expression. Like investment interest, this emotion-driven tension may build to the point where the bodymind's threshold is crossed.

The word "repression" may elicit reference to Sigmund Freud, as well as the noxious effects of bottling our emotions. Such restriction of emotional outflow is primarily a human phenomenon, as animal behavior is more instinctual and relatively unhampered by social expectations. When an animal experiences an emotion, such as anger, it will express it physically, immediately converting the emotion into action.

Humans, on the other hand, possess a more complex bodymind. Unlike animals, we often cannot immediately act upon our emotions without facing potentially serious punitive measures within our social contexts. In fact, we are regularly faced with a catch-22: we can express our emotions and pay a social toll for doing so, or we can withhold emotions to avoid the conflict but pay the price of tension, pain, or other undesirable symptoms.

Interestingly, many people experiencing pain or other bodily symptoms report that they are unaware of any strong negative emotions or stress in their lives. This process of emotional repression appears to involve a decision by the bodymind to prevent strong emotions from being consciously experienced. For reasons not entirely clear, the bodymind chooses to funnel emotional imbalances into physical symptoms.

Dr. John Sarno, a pioneer in mind-body treatments for pain, proposes that the bodymind may fear the ramifications of allowing certain strong emotions to surface to consciousness and therefore opts for a safer outlet—physical symptoms.[1] Emotions can evoke memories of past trauma which the bodymind would rather isolate then re-experience. Because this emotional repression occurs outside of our conscious awareness, those experiencing physical symptoms, such as pain, will frequently reject any proposed contribution of emotions. Though this is an understandable response, it is unfortunate in that it allows the problem to continue unabated.

Addressing Painful Emotions

Opinions differ as to the best way to address issues pertaining to subconscious emotions. Some schools of thought deny the existence of the subconscious, others simply ignore it, while others focus on it exclusively. Though the span of this book will not allow a digression into such debates, I will offer a few strategies for addressing pain involving subconscious emotions:

The Sarno Solution: Dr. Sarno believes the solution to the pain dilemma to be fairly simple, although not always easy. He emphasizes the importance of rejecting conventional explanations of pain and coming to understand pain as a result of deeply held bodymind tensions. Another aspect Dr. Sarno's pain remedy is behavior changes, such as those suggested in Appendix III.

Sarno believes his treatment approach works by foiling the bodymind's strategy of deflecting our attention from emotional issues toward physical symptoms. By exposing and deconstructing this subconscious collusion, the pain (or other symptoms) is no longer a viable strategy; the cat is out of the bag so to speak.

It is interesting to note that although Sarno's strategy does little to directly address the repressed emotions, its efficacy has been borne out in thousands of patients.[2] (I should mention that he does advocate the adjunctive use of psychotherapy for some of his patients). This seems to imply that although we all carry some degree of subconscious baggage, it doesn't have to be painful.

Expression through Words: Popularized by Sigmund Freud, "the talking cure" has been proven an effective means of improving health, though the underlying reasons for this improvement have yet to be clearly delineated. Many people realize, however, that research does not need to spell out what can be known intuitively, which is that self-expression is therapeutic. Our concept of self-expression does not need to be limited to oral communication, but may also include blogging, written letters, journaling, and so forth. Each of these allows us to express ourselves—our needs, feelings, and intentions.

A relevant study was performed at UCLA.[3] Researchers wanted to discover if the degree to which HIV-positive homosexual males were "out of the closet" affected the function of their immune systems. They found that the extent to which subjects concealed their gay identity was not simply a contributing factor, but the *most predictive factor* of the course of the disease. Those who were "fully out" had the best prognosis, while those who concealed the expression of their homosexuality showed faster progression of the disease and significantly higher rates of cancer and infectious diseases.

Another study reported that subjects who processed and recorded their deepest thoughts and feelings related to a past traumatic experience demonstrated a positive immune response. The control group, told to write only about trivial matters, showed no such response.[4]

Bodily Expression: Another route for self-expression is the body itself. Because of the intimate interplay between muscles and emotions, various forms of movement and bodywork can be effective for freeing repressed and problematic emotions; dance, art, music, and movement therapies are but examples. This may or may not involve the cathartic release of stored emotions, which is commonly reported in instances of healing.

The importance of addressing emotional content trapped in the body is supported in the research and clinical observations of Dr. Peter Levine. Levine espouses that humans (unlike other animals) often circumvent instinctual processes that serve to dispel energy following a traumatic event. His prescription involves increasing our bodily sensitivity and openness to make way for the completion of these self-healing processes (see Appendix I as a starting point for doing so).

Final Comments

Because emotions can be repressed and stored outside our conscious awareness, it can at times be difficult to determine if and how much they are contributing to a painful problem. This notwithstanding, implementing strategies for dealing with strong emotions frequently results in reduced pain. It may help to think of the bodymind as comparable to a ledger of pluses and minuses, so that progress in one arena, such as emotions, can lead to a significant improvement in your experience as a whole.

8

FINDING MEANING

"You've wandered all over and finally realized that you never found what you were after: how to live" —Marcus Aurelius

In earlier chapters, we discussed the inconsistent relationship between bodily abnormalities and pain, as one person may encounter tremendous pain without injury, while another may report minimal pain despite serious injury. To make sense of this apparent conundrum, we learned the necessity of viewing pain in its broader contexts. Pain does not exist in a bodily vacuum, but impacts relationships, self-identity, and personal aspirations. When pain is perceived as hindering these important qualities of life, we may feel we are "suffering."

Unfortunately, our society and medical system have attempted to treat pain while downplaying suffering, effectively divorcing the pain from its contexts. People are subjected to innumerable tests and procedures which often fail to accurately identify the origin of the problem. Such inadequacy in measuring or explaining suffering can evoke feelings of invalidation, hopelessness, confusion, frustration, or some combination thereof. The fact is that in many cases, pain cannot be curtailed if its human context is ignored.

In this chapter, we will explore these issues from a few different angles. First, we will examine the foundational role of meaning in human life. This will be followed by further discussion of the interrelatedness of pain, meaning, and suffering. We will conclude by articulating ways of investing our experiences, painful or otherwise, with greater meaning and purpose. My hope is that this chapter will facilitate some semblance of peace with your current circumstances, however they may appear.

The Foundational Role of Meaning in Human Life

Perhaps, at some point in your life's journey, you have wrestled with some of the following questions: What is the meaning of life? What is the purpose of *my* life? What is missing from my life? These are some of the most ubiquitous and deeply felt questions of humanity, fully occupying the attention of innumerable sages, philosophers, and reformers throughout history. The fact remains that we simply cannot avoid looking for meaning, and doing so in all arenas of life.

Even the mundane can be construed as meaningful. Eating a piece of food has meaning in the sense of knowing you will not go hungry that day. A smile from a stranger may be interpreted as "I'm likeable" or "She's in a good mood." When things are not going so well, such as in the classic children's book *Alexander & the Terrible, Horrible, No Good, Very Bad Day*, we want to know why: Why does everything seem to be going wrong today? What did I do to deserve this?

Whenever we ask such questions and try to understand our experiences, we are in fact seeking meaning. This occurs both consciously and subconsciously, perhaps even when we are dreaming. In short, the quest for meaning permeates the world of human endeavors.

Values are closely related to meaning. In our culture, we hear talk about "family values" or at the supermarket, "great values." More generally, values embody what we interpret to be good, beautiful, or desirable. Some values are universal—the value of food, shelter, clothing, relationships, etc.—whereas others are more individualized, such as musical preference, political preferences, etc.

Despite the specific content of each of our values, they influence our decisions at every step. What we eat, what we wear, how we interact with others, where we live and shop—these are all value-based judgments. Like meaning-seeking, we cannot escape valuation.

When we regard an activity as valuable and decide to pursue it, we can be said to be acting "purposefully." Purpose exists on both large and small scales. Deciding to get out of bed in the morning is purposeful, just as declaring your intent to become president. Often, however, smaller purposes are subservient to grander life purposes. For instance, you may decide to get out of bed *so that* you can pursue your presidential aspirations. So when people discuss "purpose," they often are referring to an overarching purpose, such as the "What do you want to be when you grow up?" notion. These grand purposes are fueled by our values, interests, and sense of identity, serving as attractors for our personal decisions and development.

The final concept related to this discussion is that of authenticity. A life can said to be authentic when a person's behavior is consistent with his or her purpose and values. This extends to all areas of life, including choices of mate, work, and leisure activities. If your behavior contradicts your values, a sense of uneasiness, tension, or guilt may arise. The experience of "conscience" or "conviction" is derived from such experiences. As a result of the discomfort that may arise from inauthentic action, most people, knowingly or not, strive to act authentically.

Clearly, all of these concepts, ultimately rooted in meaning, are foundational to our lives. It should therefore come as no surprise that they also play a critical role in our pain experiences. Next, we will discuss this important interplay of pain, meaning, and suffering.

Pain, Meaning, & Suffering

Pain is invested with meaning on a number of levels, spanning from the slightest twinge to the life-altering spiral of chronic pain. In some instances, the intent of pain is immediately obvious, such as when touching a hot stove. In others, ambiguity may provoke interrogation of the pain experience: Why is this happening? What did I do to deserve this? How could I have prevented it? It is these instances—when pain seems random, meaningless, and undeserved—that are most difficult to endure and foment the most suffering.

A well-known account of such struggles is the biblical story of Job. Job is a story about suffering, a story which embodies the question: How much pain, evil, and suffering can a single person withstand before he will "curse God and die?"

Despite the hyperbolic nature of Job's suffering, the story effectively highlights some of the central issues relating pain, suffering, and meaning. When Job is robbed of his possessions and family, he finds himself alone in his struggles. Though he is left with a few friends, they struggle to comprehend his pain or his resultant actions.

As the tragedy continues, Job's attention is gradually turned away from the outer world and toward his inner struggle for meaning. He is compelled to examine spiritual and emotional issues—a sort of tug-of-war for his soul. Several hundred years later, Jesus, in the climax of his suffering, expressed a similar flood of loneliness and struggle in his urgent cry "Why have you forsaken me?"

As in the accounts of Job and Jesus, the experience of pain, particularly chronic pain, invokes a sense of isolation. In her book, *The Body in Pain*, Elaine Scarry emphasizes the inexpressibility of pain and the resultant difficulty of comprehending another's experience; regardless of how hard we may try, we can never *fully* understand. The problem of pain is exacerbated by the absence of social and emotional support, as expressions of suffering fall on deaf ears.

With or without an outlet for its expression, suffering may inspire inner examination and spiritual reflection: How can I make sense of this pain? How can I take what is left in my life and make the most of it? Should I give up or fight? Or, more broadly: How does my current experience fit with my life story as a whole? For those who partake in such inner dialogue, a shift in thinking often transpires, as the previous view of self and the world no longer appears appropriate and is replaced by one that is more congruent and useful.[1]

Returning to our example of Job, what remains once life as we know it is stripped away? What kernel of our humanity is impervious to our physical circumstances? Under dire circumstances such as these, some may find religion, while others may lose it. What all will attempt to find, however, is some semblance of meaning. Chronic pain or serious illness quickly sharpens and redirects our focus toward our uniquely human need for meaning.

In his book, *Man's Search for Meaning,* psychologist Victor Frankl describes his experience as a prisoner in a Nazi concentration camp. One of Frankl's most salient observations detailed how factors such as strength and muscularity failed to account for who survived amid the horrific and dehumanizing circumstances. Instead, Frankl noted that the sanity and survival of the prisoners depended on their ability to hold to something that could not be destroyed: "The prisoner who had lost faith in the future—his future—was doomed. With loss of belief in the future, one also lost his spiritual hold, allowing himself to acquiesce to mental and physical decay."[2] Again, we find similar sentiments echoed in words ascribed to Jesus: "Do not be afraid of those who kill the body but cannot kill the soul."[3]

To the extent that pain engenders inner reflection and a deepened sense of meaning, it can be said to be therapeutic. Dr. Mitchell Smolkin, in his book *Understanding Pain,* describes the concept of "therapeutic ratio," which suggests that every type of experience, including pain, can be viewed on a continuum that spans from detrimental to helpful. Though this ratio varies with the individual, it implies that sustaining some amount of pain can be beneficial for facilitating personal growth.

Smolkin's suggestion that pain may possess some positive value makes a degree of sense in light of our earlier discussion of bodymind balance. This may be especially true in newer onsets of pain, which can serve to indicate bodymind imbalance and may inspire beneficial life changes. As the duration of pain extends into several months or years, however, it becomes more deeply engrained into the bodymind, thereby diminishing its effectiveness as an accurate signifier of imbalance. Thus, finding hope or meaning in the trenches of chronic pain can become increasingly difficult. This appears especially true for those who remained focused on finding a medical cure, which serves as a distraction from accessing potent inner resources.

Purpose in Life & Work

Purpose and meaning are integral to life satisfaction, health, and longevity. Unfortunately, it seems that our passion for life—what Wilhem Reich referred to as "life energy"—often devolves to a state of apathy once our school days are over. It's as though we have come to expect life's major challenges and curiosities to end once we reach adulthood. We forget how to wonder about our life journeys, believing that we've already arrived at the answers to all the burning questions (e.g. – Where will I work? Who will I marry? Etc.). When this occurs, our lives can become regimented and predictable, devoid of meaningful engagement, curiosity, and spontaneity.

Those who avoid falling victim to the apathetic life are less likely to succumb to ill health. It seems that possessing a passion for life, explicit or otherwise, powerfully dictates the direction of our bodily processes. In this sense, health is not merely related to fewer hardships, but involves the presence of an active and vital current of engagement.

One important conduit for purposeful activity is work, whether done for income or otherwise. In ideal circumstances, a person's work will integrate his or her skills, values, and interests, while providing a sense of purposeful engagement. This reminds me of the book entitled *Do What You Are*, which highlights the importance of our preferences and abilities with respect to our vocational selection. When this is done carefully, work will often not feel like work, since perception of time and effort are lost in the flow of the activity.

As an illustration, you may have noticed an increased sense of vitality on the weekends, even after working all day in the yard or vigorously pursuing a favorite pastime. This can be attributed to the fact that your bodymind responds favorably when performing enjoyable work, generating energy even in the midst of concentrated activity.

One way of improving your life is to actively work toward identifying or developing your preferred vocation. I am not suggesting an immediate job change, but a *process* of exploration, examination, and experimentation, both within and outside your present job. For many people, their ideal work comes only after years of discovery and growth in a variety of circumstances.

If you are dissatisfied with your current work life, there are other factors to consider as well. For example, if you hesitate to change jobs because of financial concerns, you may wish to reconsider what possessions are actually required to meet your basic needs and attempt to downsize accordingly. Sometimes, maintaining a certain standard of living requires a forfeiture of leisure time and causes more strain than pleasure. Upon consideration, you may decide that such a lifestyle is not worth the additional time and stress.

Another consideration is the work that you perform around the house. If you feel like you are always pressed for time and unable to enjoy your favorite pastimes, you may wish to question the tasks that you believe to be mandatory. Ask yourself why you do the things you do. Is it because the task really needs to be done, or are you simply performing it out of habit or convention? Things such as washing the car, weeding the yard, or other tasks that are not truly necessary may be causing you unneeded stress. For me, I've found that reducing the things on my "must do" list has significantly freed my schedule for the pursuit of my core passions.

Closing Thoughts

Many aspects of life are not easy or comfortable. We don't live in a utopian world and things often seem unfair or unreasonable. The fact that life can be replete with hardships is often referred to as "the human condition." Despite the inherent challenges of life, we also possess unique abilities and options, such as the freedom to formulate our life course and experiences.

If you are suffering with pain, you have choices. If you conclude that your health and life will never improve, that is one choice. But there are others. No matter your stage in life, I encourage you to try to make the most of it. You may even find yourself pleasantly surprised.

FINISHING TOUCHES

As discussed in Chapter 3, in order to flourish, our bodymind must remain balanced within certain parameters. In this section, I summarize what I believe to be among the most important recommendations for restoring balance and reducing pain. After doing so, we will look at a case study for purposes of illustration and application.

Before reviewing our key recommendations, I wanted to provide a pictorial representation of various factors which may contribute to pain. The following figure can serve as a reminder of the multi-factorial nature of pain, as well as the fact that pain can be addressed through a variety of different means. Remember, pain is context-dependent and will change when surrounding factors are altered.

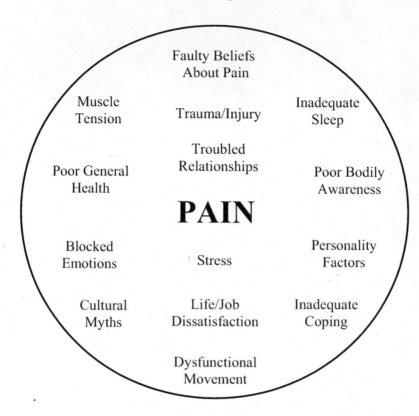

With this picture of pain in mind, let's proceed by highlighting some of the recommendations presented in earlier chapters. Please do not feel that you have to tackle them all at once. Instead, undertake one at a time, being sure to notice the improvement that results from even the simplest of changes. Make it a point to consistently remind yourself of your intentions and use this book as a source of regular reinforcement and encouragement. Remember, it is sometimes best to focus your efforts on restoring balance with your life circumstances, as the bodymind specializes in healing itself once obstacles are removed. What follows is an expanded version of our

CEO acronym. I encourage you to take responsibility as the CEO of your health and life.

Change your thoughts and behavior toward pain:

- *Expand your understanding of pain, eliminate erroneous beliefs, accept responsibility for your health, and cultivate a positive outlook:* These sentiments are really the heart of this book. It is particularly important to understand the role of beliefs, expectations, and emotions with respect to pain. The body-machine story must be reevaluated in light of this broader and more comprehensive framework. We must repudiate notions such as "I have a bad back" and recognize the harm that results from such fatalistic thinking. Learning to become more optimistic, grateful, and hopeful is also indispensable to our health (see Appendix II).

- *Think critically about medical advice and diagnoses:* This was addressed in Chapters 4 and 5 and suggests that we need to actively participate in gathering information and making decisions about our health.

- *Restore movement, return to normal activities, and overcome fear-avoidance behavior:* If you are not moving normally, pain will often continue, even if the tissues are healed. Overcoming fear-avoidance, an important contributor to chronic pain, is tackled in Appendix III.

Enhance your bodily awareness:

- *Increase your sensitivity and understanding of your body:* Both animals and indigenous peoples can sense and escape natural disasters through their awareness and respect for their instincts and intuition. Unfortunately, many of us have no more than a dulled awareness of our bodies and have lost the ability to sense its promptings. By increasing your bodily knowledge and awareness, you can acquire important information for restoring bodymind balance and reducing pain. Enhancing your awareness of your breathing, tension, sensations, and movements are important aspects of this learning process. I have included some introductory activities for initiating this process in Appendix I.

Overhaul other aspects of your health and life:

- *Recognize the critical role of stress and emotions (both conscious and unconscious) in painful problems:* Both intense short-term and more systemic long-term stress can precipitate pain, as can repressed emotions. As indicated in Chapter 3, the bodymind provides us with warning signs that precede the crossing of its threshold. In many cases, these signs include feelings of stress or tension, which should be addressed to allow balance to be restored.

- *Express yourself authentically and engage in meaningful pursuits:* This involves the authentic expression of emotions, as well as engaging in work, relationships, movement, and creative endeavors that match your inner desires. It seems that the more we opt to compromise our authenticity, the greater risk we run for inner conflict, pain, and other health problems.

- *Take steps toward improving your general health, including reducing body weight and increasing physical activity:* You are probably aware of the importance of bettering your general health, but you may not have recognized its ramifications for your pain.

- *Open your heart and connect to something beyond yourself:* Intimate relationships, religion/spirituality, and close-knit communities provide a context for authentic self-expression, shared meaning and values, and fostering hope.

A Case Study Application

Lori came to me hoping that I could help her with her chronic back pain. Though the pain had been most excruciating and persistent in the left side of her lower back and thigh, she reported that it had recently spread to her right hip and buttock. She described how the pain worsened as the day progressed, especially if she engaged in any form of physical activity. As a result of her disability, she experienced feelings of depression and hopelessness, desperate to return to her former way of life.

Lori indicated that the pain had begun about three years prior, approximately two years into her job as a production worker. She recalled bending to pick up a part—something she did on a daily basis—when she suddenly experienced what felt like a knife thrust into her lower back. After seeing the company physician, she was referred for a course of physical therapy.

Though she experienced temporary relief with therapy treatments, the pain always seemed to return with a vengeance, making it difficult for her to think about anything else. The doctor recommended she undergo an MRI, but findings were inconclusive. It revealed a lumbar disc protruding to the right, but most of her pain had been on the left. Despite this, she proceeded to have surgery, hoping that fixing the disc would also fix the pain.

Not surprisingly, the surgery failed, along with a second one, to correct the problem. Lori reported that she had felt pretty good for about a week afterward, but the pain slowly returned, to the point where it seemed worse than prior to the operations. Beyond surgery, she tried other treatments such as chiropractic, a special type of mattress for her bed, and a variety of different herbal remedies and medications. When I asked her if she had seen a counselor or psychotherapist, she said that she had considered it, but didn't think it would have done much good. After all, pain—physical pain—was her problem.

In order to get a better sense of the context of her pain, I asked Lori to recall some of her life circumstances at the time. She remembered going through a particularly difficult period, including the loss of a loved one, a pending divorce, as well as other poignant stressors. We discussed the role that these factors may have played in contributing to imbalance in her bodymind, as well as the possibility that her injury at work was merely the last straw. Over time, she was able to acknowledge the role of stress and strong emotions in both the initiation and continuance of her pain.

In addition to understanding the broader causes of her pain, it was necessary for us to address her fears relating to pain, movement, and activity. After all, she had grown tired of pain and was doing all she possibly could to try to avoid it. The first step in altering these fears involved teaching her how to relax her bodymind.

Due to the long-standing nature of her pain, Lori was actually incapable of fully relaxing when we first began; there was too much tension and fear engrained in her physiology. However, with a little guidance and experimentation with her positioning and breathing, she learned that relaxation was something she could achieve. This was actually a huge boost of confidence for her, as she previously felt helpless with respect to her anxiety and muscle tension.

Once she had acquired the ability to fully relax, I helped her to initiate very slow and gentle movements, while encouraging her to maintain a relaxed state while moving. This was difficult at first, as she tended to revert to her old patterns of tension, fearing the pain might worsen. Despite this, she gradually learned to move in a relaxed fashion. Her range of motion improved significantly, while her fear of pain was greatly reduced. In fact, she discovered that her pain sensations, without the added fear and tension, were rather benign and tolerable. With her newfound ability to relax and move more freely, I encouraged her to increase her activity levels at home and begin a walking regimen. Though still painful at times, she slowly increased her walking distance and began tackling much of the housework she had for so long avoided.

Lori reported difficulty letting go of her feelings of anger, contempt, and shame that surrounded her divorce. Though she remained uninterested in pursuing psychotherapy, I encouraged her to discover an outlet for her emotions. After considering some suggestions, she decided to reinitiate an activity she had loved as a kid, journaling. She found that journaling helped her to organize her thoughts and make some sense of her feelings. In the process, she began to contemplate where she wanted to go with her life, including the possibility of taking some college classes.

After about three months of working intermittently with Lori, she looked like a new person. Her posture had improved, she displayed new life in her eyes, and she moved with a sense of confidence and vigor. Although she disliked spending three years of her life in chronic pain, she reported that the process of her recovery had kindled newfound strength and self-knowledge that she may not have encountered otherwise. Her experience with pain, though incredibly trying, had given her a fresh perspective on life.

POSTSCRIPT

In the first chapter of the book, I highlighted the fact that we are story-telling creatures and that our stories impact our health and well-being. Particularly, it is clear that some stories, including those about pain, are not as accurate or beneficial as others. Hopefully, this book has provided you with some basic ingredients for constructing a more coherent and useful story.

Though it is true that we may never fully comprehend our inherent potential for healing and growth, transformation begins with an attitude of openness and positive expectation. If you are struggling with your health, I especially challenge you to embrace this vision for transformation. You may choose to pursue this through further reading, bodywork, conversation, introspection, self-experimentation, or a variety of other means. At minimum, I hope you realize that you no longer need to be bound by a diagnosis or anyone else's opinion about your condition.

You can heal. Even if your physical healing was to remain incomplete, you can still heal mentally, emotionally, and spiritually; if you do only that, I can assure you that your physical maladies will seem less detrimental. I encourage you to make the choice to take back your life, recover your spirit, and make peace with yourself and your circumstances.

Thank you so much for reading and joining me on this exciting journey of *Re-Thinking Pain.* My hope is that the thoughts in this book have resonated as authentic and hopeful, inspiring renewal in your mind, body, and spirit.

Chapter Notes

Complete references can be found in the *Sources* section.

Introduction

1. Gatchel RJ. *Clinical Essentials of Pain Management.*
2. Morris D. *Illness and Culture in the Postmodern Age.*
3. Kosambi DD. "Living Prehistory in India."
4. Bayer T, Baer P, & Charles E. "Situational and Psychophysiological Factors in Psychologically Induced Pain."
5. In attempting to understand health and illness, it seems necessary to acknowledge the valid contributions of both science and intuition. The fact that analytic and holistic thought are essential to human knowing is supported by research into the workings of the brain. Though specific brain functions are rarely confined to a single area of the brain, scientists have discovered that the brain's two hemispheres tend to have specialized functions. The right hemisphere of the brain, sometimes called the right brain, is thought to be largely responsible for phenomena such as mental images, intuition, and non-linear (i.e., "all at once") knowing. It incorporates rapid, subconscious processes, allowing us to see the whole picture quickly without conscious thinking or deliberate analysis. This hemisphere could be conceptualized as acting more primitively (not in a bad or inferior sense) and may be difficult to differentiate from "gut instincts."

   In contrast, the left hemisphere, or left brain, tends to be more instrumental in language, analysis, logic, and linear cause-effect reasoning. Left-brain processes may take significantly longer than those of the right, as conscious deliberation can at times be painstakingly slow. Despite this, the left brain is often mistakenly heralded as more effective or more intelligent than its right-brain counterpart, a fallacy which is nicely countered in Malcolm Gladwell's *Blink: The Power of Thinking Without Thinking*. Without intuition, we would have never survived long enough to develop the culture and language necessary for what we now recognize as conscious, left-brain thought.

Chapter 2

1. Gatchel RJ. *Clinical Essentials of Pain Management.*
2. Benson H. *Timeless Healing: The Power and Biology of Belief.*
3. Kleinman A. *Rethinking Psychiatry.*
4. Louser JD. "Low Back Pain."
5. Melzack R, Wall PD, & Ty TC. "Acute Pain in an Emergency Clinic: Latency of Onset and Descriptor Patterns Related to Different Injuries."
6. Borenstein DJ, et al. "The Value of Magnetic Resonance Imaging of the Lumbar Spine to Predict Low-Back Pain in Asymptomatic Subjects"; Gatchel RJ & Turk DC, eds. *Psychosocial Factors in Pain*; Jensen MC, et al. "Magnetic Resonance Imaging of the Lumbar Spine in People without Back Pain."; Sarno J. *The Mindbody Prescription*; Siegel RD, et al. *Back Sense.*
7. Fox AJ, et al. "Myelographic Cervical Nerve Root Deformities."
8. Borenstein DJ, et al. "The Value of Magnetic Resonance Imaging of the Lumbar Spine to Predict Low-Back Pain in Asymptomatic Subjects"; Gatchel RJ & Turk DC, eds. *Psychosocial Factors in Pain*; Jensen MC, et al. "Magnetic Resonance Imaging of the Lumbar Spine in People without Back Pain."; Sarno J. *The Mindbody Prescription*; Siegel RD, et al. *Back Sense.*

9. Borenstein DJ, et al. "The Value of Magnetic Resonance Imaging of the Lumbar Spine to Predict Low-Back Pain in Asymptomatic Subjects."

10. Kleinman A. *Rethinking Psychiatry.*

11. Gatchel RJ & Turk DC, eds. *Psychosocial Factors in Pain*; Pincus T, et al. "A Systematic Review of Psychological Factors as Predictors of Chronicity/Disability in Prospective Cohorts of Low Back Pain."; Williams RA, et al. "The Contribution of Job Satisfaction to the Transition from Acute to Chronic Low Back Pain."

12. Bigos SJ, et al. "A Prospective Study of Work Perceptions and Psychosocial Factors Affecting the Reporting of a Back Injury."

13. Gatchel RJ & Turk DC, eds. *Psychosocial Factors in Pain*; Williams RA, et al. "The Contribution of Job Satisfaction to the Transition from Acute to Chronic Low Back Pain."

14. Carron H, DeGood D, & Tait R. "A Comparison of Low Back Pain Patients in the United States and New Zealand: Psychological and Economic Factors Affecting Severity and Disability."

15. Brena SF, Sanders SH, & Motoyama H. "American and Japanese Low Back Pain Patients: Cross-Cultural Similarities and Differences."

16. Sanders SH, et al. "Chronic Low Back Pain Patients around the World: Cross Cultural Similarities and Differences."

17. Shrader H, et al. "Natural Evolution of Late Whiplash Syndrome Outside the Medicolegal Context."

18. Kleinman A. *Rethinking Psychiatry.*

19. Siegel, et al. *Back Sense.*

20. Bogduk N. "Management of Chronic Low Back Pain."

21. Dimond EG, Kittle CF, & Crockett JE. "Comparison of Internal Mammary Ligation and Sham Operation for Angina Pectoris."; Moseley, et al. "A Controlled Trial of Arthroscopic Surgery for Osteoarthritis of the Knee."

22. Spangforte EV. "The Lumbar Disk Herniation: A Computer-Aided Analysis of 2504 Operations."

23. Bogduk N. "Management of Chronic Low Back Pain."

24. Illich I. *Medical Nemesis.*

25. Gatchel RJ & Turk DC, eds. *Psychosocial Factors in Pain.*

Chapter 3

1. Aposhyan S. *Natural Intelligence*; Lipton B. *The Biology of Belief*; Pert C. *Molecules of Emotion.*

2. Though we tend to conceptualize our bodily experiences as involving a simple signal from one part of the body to the brain (such as the stomach telling the brain when it is empty), things are actually more complex than that. In fact, the bodymind is constantly evaluating huge amounts of input from both its internal and external environments. This includes information about movement, pressure, temperature (both internal and external), auditory and visual input, chemical balances, beliefs, emotions, memories, etc. If we were required to handle all of this information in our *conscious* minds, we would probably experience information overload, finding ourselves overwhelmed and incompetent for negotiating such a task. Fortunately, this information is filtered and sorted subconsciously, a process which determines what is most important for us to consciously experience at any particular moment.

3. Wall PD. *Pain: The Science of Suffering.*

4. Actually, the ability of seemingly small shifts to induce rapid and dramatic changes throughout an entire system is supported by studies of complex physical systems (e.g. - chaos theory).

5. The framework outlined in this chapter remains quite general in that it does not specify what type of pain may result following the crossing of the threshold. For clarification, I will defer to the concept of "diathesis-stress" (Gatchel & Turk, eds. *Psychosocial Factors in Pain*. pp. 249-256), which suggests that individuals possess vulnerability to the development of certain types of pain or illness. Though many of us have common areas of vulnerability (e.g. – the low back), variability exists across individuals and cultures. The "stress" portion of the model indicates that such vulnerabilities translate to illness upon the addition of further imbalance to the system. This is quite similar to my concept of threshold. For more on the integral role of stress in crossing the bodymind threshold, see Chapter 6.

Chapter 4

1. In my estimation, comparing the longevity, health, and healing capacities of humans with that of other animals provides some of the most compelling evidence for acknowledging the role of psycho-cultural factors in human illness. If we share some 99% of our DNA with chimpanzees, we must ask ourselves how we differ and why we are more prone to chronic illness. The answer in both cases appears to involve, among other things, psycho-cultural factors. Though there is some degree of difference in health and longevity within other animal species, it is nowhere near the variation that we regularly witness in humans. Much of this variation may be attributed to the plasticity of the human nervous system, which is more open to environmental shaping than that of our primate ancestors. As I

discuss in Chapter 5, the major adaptations that are incurred during early nurturing can be positive or negative. In cases of poor nurturing, the formation of an aberrant physiology and psychology can contribute to ill health throughout life, including premature aging and death.

2. Houston J. *Life Force*, p. 245.

3. Martin P. *The Healing Mind.*

4. Sapolsky RM. *Why Zebras Don't Get Ulcers.*

5. Achterberg J. *Imagery in Healing.*

6. Hall E & Haydel M. "Conversion Disorder Presenting as Hemiplegia and Hemianesthesia with Loss of Neurologic Reflexes: A Case Report."

7. See Pengel LHM, et al. "Acute Low Back Pain: Systematic Review of Its Prognosis."; Waddell G. *The Back Pain Revolution.*

8. See Achterberg J. *Imagery in Healing.*

9. Ibid.

10. Brody H. *The Placebo Response.*

11. Kleinman A. *Rethinking Psychiatry*; Schlitz M & Amorok T, eds. *Consciousness and Healing.*

12. Lipton B. *The Biology of Belief.*

13. Moseley B, et al. "A Controlled Trial of Arthroscopic Surgery for Osteoarthritis of the Knee."

14. See Lipton B, *The Biology of Belief*, p. 139.

15. Fritz JM, George SZ, & Delito A. "The Role of Fear-Avoidance Beliefs in Acute Low Back Pain: Relationships with Current and Future Disability and Work Status."

16. Ibid.

17. A primary factor contributing to the difficulty of overcoming fear-avoidance is its inherently self-reinforcing nature. Let's say that I have a fear of bending at the waist. Occasionally, I might decide to

test this behavior to see if my fear of pain is actually justified. When doing so, it is likely that I will experience the expected pain. Why is this the case? A couple reasons come to mind. First, the fear of the behavior may become a self-fulfilling prophecy, as anticipated pain serves to prime the bodymind to experience it. Second, fear of movement often results in an exaggerated tensing of muscles upon movement which may increase the likelihood of experiencing pain. Thus, when pain occurs with such testing, fear-avoidance beliefs are strengthened and testing becomes less frequent. In reality, the activity might not be so painful if expectations were different.

18. See Achterberg J. *Imagery in Healing.*
19. Levine P. *Waking the Tiger: Healing Trauma.*

Chapter 5

1. See Dychtwald K. *Bodymind*; Arraj J. *Tracking the Elusive Human Volume II.* Arraj provides a fascinating treatment of the pioneering work of W.H. Sheldon, most famous for his coining of three somatotypes (body types): ectomorphic, mesomorphic, and endomorphic. What many have overlooked and Arraj brings to the forefront, is Sheldon's data and discussion connecting physique and temperament. If nothing else, it makes for an interesting read.
2. Gladwell, M. *Blink: The Power of Thinking Without Thinking.*
3. Sarno J. *The Mindbody Prescription*; Siegel RD, et al. *Back Sense.*
4. See Butler D. *The Sensitive Nervous System.*
5. Symonds TL, et al. "Absence Resulting from Low Back Trouble Can Be Reduced by Psychosocial Intervention at the Work Place."
6. Ibid.
7. Butler D. *The Sensitive Nervous System.*

8. Nicklas BJ, You T, & Pahor M. "Behavioral Treatment for Chronic Systemic Inflammation: Effects of Dietary Weight Loss and Exercise."

9. Ibid.

10. Ibid.

11. See Butler D. *The Sensitive Nervous System.*

12. Ibid.

13. Cymet TC & Sinkov V. "Does Long-Distance Running Cause Osteoarthritis?"

14. Ibid.

15. Fries JF, et al. "Running and the Development of Disability with Age."

16. For those interested in thought-provoking commentary on overuse/repetitive stress injuries, I encourage you to peruse *Repetitive Stress Injury: Diagnosis or Self-Fulfilling Prophecy?* (Szabo & King) and *Neurosis in the Workplace* (Lucire). In these reports, the authors emphasize that the current prevalence of workplace-related disorders has been largely fostered through societal expectations and public policy, rather than an increase in physical injuries. In other words, our medical/legal system, in its current form, provides a socially and legally acceptable space for these types of problems to arise and flourish, leading to greater numbers of health complaints. As medical anthropologist Yolande Lucire writes, many physicians have come to abide by the axiom that *"judging a sick person to be well is more important to avoid than judging a well person to be sick."* Granted, this is in part (perhaps largely) due to the fear of legal action should an actual disease diagnosis be missed. Nevertheless, one must question if this axiom is actually not more injurious than good, as conflating symptoms of life distress with medical disease has led to greater incidence of chronic illness and disability.

The fact that culture and its institutions influence the incidence and characteristics of illness is the manifesto of eminent Harvard anthropologist-physician Arthur Kleinman. In his books, *Rethinking Psychiatry* and *Writing at the Margin*, Kleinman convincingly demonstrates that any particular culture and medical system serve to shape the nature and expression of illness in its constituents. In America, it is not surprising that the notion of overuse injury has proliferated within the predominant cultural story of the body-machine. It also seems likely that the emergence of work-related pain complaints was inadvertently fostered by an otherwise well-intended campaign for worker rights, protection, and safety. Out of this climate of concern arose the field of ergonomics, which has not significantly reduced the prevalence of claims, despite improvements in worker comfort (Szabo & King).

17. Bigos SJ, et al. "A Prospective Study of Work Perceptions and Psychosocial Factors Affecting the Reporting of a Back Injury."; Gatchel RJ & Turk DC, eds. *Psychosocial Factors in Pain*; Pincus, et al. "A Systematic Review of Psychological Factors as Predictors of Chronicity/Disability in Prospective Cohorts of Low Back Pain."; Williams RA, et al. "The Contribution of Job Satisfaction to the Transition from Acute to Chronic Low Back Pain."

It is also interesting to note that the anatomical locations involved in many of these syndromes are synonymous with the tender points used for diagnosing fibromyalgia, a condition which appears to have strong psychosocial underpinnings. Thus, in cohort with Dr. John Sarno, I suspect that similar underlying processes may be at work in many of cases of work-related pain.

18. Feldenkrais M. *The Elusive Obvious*.

19. Kepner J. *Body Process*.

20. Ibid.

Chapter 6

1. Kleinman A. *Rethinking Psychiatry.*
2. Ibid.
3. Sarno J. *The Mindbody Prescription.*
4. An onset of pain or illness may effectively force you to leave stressful circumstances or to seek social support, actions which you may not have taken otherwise. Social support provides a sense that one's burdens are being shared, thereby lowering the perceived level of stress and reducing imbalance. It also mitigates fear about the future, as there seems to be a sort of "strength in numbers" in the human psyche.
5. Brody H. *The Placebo Response.*
6. Chatterjee C. "Stop the Pain."; Gatchel RJ. *Clinical Essentials of Pain Management* ; Wilber K. *Integral Psychology.*
7. Chatterjee C.
8. Prinz P. "Sleep, Appetite, and Obesity—What is the Link?"
9. Ghaly M & Teplitz D. "The Biologic Effects of Grounding the Human Body During Sleep by Cortisol Levels and Subjective Reports of Sleep, Pain, and Stress."
10. Ibid.
11. Newth S & Delongis A. "Individual Differences, Mood, and Coping with Chronic Pain in Rheumatoid Arthritis: A Daily Process Analysis."
12. Lounsbury JW, et al. "Personality, Career Satisfaction, and Life Satisfaction."
13. Boddeker I & Stemmler G. "Who Responds How and When to Anger? The Assessment of Actual Anger Response Styles and Their Relation to Personality."
14. Ibid.

15. Spiegal D, et al. "Effect of Psychosocial Treatment on Survival of Patients with Metastatic Breast Cancer."
16. Ibid.

Chapter 7

1. Sarno J. *The Mindbody Prescription.*
2. Ibid.
3. Cole S, et al. "Elevated Physical Health Risk among Gay Men Who Conceal Their Homosexual Identity."
4. Pennebaker JW. "Confession, Inhibition, and Disease."

Chapter 8

1. Smolkin MT. *Understanding Pain: Interpretation and Philosophy.*
2. Frankl V. *Man's Search for Meaning.*
3. Matthew 10:28 (NIV)

I

ENHANCING YOUR BODILY AWARENESS

"Lose your mind and come to your senses."—Fritz Perl

This appendix is designed to elaborate on the second component of our CEO acronym: "Enhance your bodily awareness." By nature, this component is not as easily described as the others, since it is best understood through experience. It is for this reason that I have included some sample exercises below.

Before describing some bodily awareness exercises, I wanted to highlight some of their fundamental ingredients: awareness, breath, movement, relaxation, and touch. Awareness appears to be the most vital component, as movement, breathing, or relaxation alone may do little to facilitate a more sensitive, integrated bodymind. Earlier, we touched on the importance of diaphragmatic breathing, which I suggested as an important component for decreasing stress and increasing bodily awareness. Though there are a myriad of ways to incorporate breath when working with your body, its most critical contributions seem to involve inducing relaxation and serving as a center for awareness. For example, when working with my body, if I encounter an area of tightness, pain, or restriction, I will often pause, focus on my breathing, and allow the relaxation that accompanies each exhalation to slowly dissolve the tension. Movement is another great way to reduce tension and increase bodily awareness (discussed below), as is touch (e.g. - self-massage).

There is no right or wrong way to enhance your bodily awareness. Your personal preferences will depend largely on your personality as well as your current level of familiarity with your body and its workings. From the following exercises, please feel free to pick and choose what you like. *You may wish to consult with your physician before you begin.* Remember, the point isn't to follow a script, but to listen, learn, and explore your body. Over time, I am confident that you will reap great rewards for doing so, as I have encountered personally and professionally.

1) Introductory Awareness Exercise: Lie or sit with your eyes gently closed, assuming a comfortable, relaxed position. Bring your attention to how your body feels as a whole. Notice the subtle buzz or vibration that is present throughout. Over time, bring your focus to different aspects of your body. Notice your breathing and the nature of your inhalation and exhalation rhythms. How does your body feel as you observe your breathing? Are you fully relaxed or do some areas of tension remain? Be sure to survey your facial muscles, which often signal whether the rest of your body is fully relaxed. If you notice tension, bring your attention to those areas and allow the muscles to release (initiating small, slow oscillating movements may help you learn how your muscles work and what is necessary to relax them). As you transition toward deeper relaxation (which may seem difficult at first), simply enjoy the experience of balance and wholeness. Throughout the process, commemorate the fact that simply experiencing your own bodymind can be so pleasurable.

While practicing, it is normal to notice your mind wandering. Try not to become frustrated (it happens to everybody!), but simply return to your intended focus. Remember, part of awareness is noticing what is happening with your thoughts, so the realization that your mind wandering is actually part of your awareness education.

2) Getting to Know Your Pain: If you are experiencing pain in a certain area, you may wish to try the following: Start by attaining a comfortable position so you can relax and focus, using pillows or other props as needed. Once you are comfortable and relaxed, bring your full awareness to the painful area. Attempt to get inside of it and learn everything about it that you can. Try to comprehend what it really feels like throughout the region. Attend to the surface level, then move deeper. Notice any pulsations, movements, or sensations that are present. Try to avoid fearing the pain or judging it as "bad," simply observe with as little emotion or fear as possible. Part of learning about the area is understanding what it feels like when you move it. When doing so, start with slow, subtle movements, usually with your eyes closed so that you can fully capture how it feels. As you learn what the area feels like apart from fear, you will learn to better tolerate and accept your bodily sensations. Believe it or not, with practice, you will begin to view the pain as less concerning, as something that you do not need to fear or avoid. You can also try dispersing the pain, picturing it moving out of the area and out of your body.

3) Awareness through Movement Exercise: Awareness can be cultivated by maintaining awareness while moving. In other words, if you learn to pay attention to how your body movements feel as you move, you will become more aware of your bodymind in general and become more competent in satisfying its needs (see Chapter 3).

Dr. Moshe Feldenkrais emphasized that his awareness through movement exercises were not intended as therapy per se, but as a means of learning and increasing one's potential. Learning, in his conception, engendered new possibilities for both mind and body, which he believed to be critical to optimal living. Without options, we cannot adapt to a changing world, which eventually may precipitate pain or illness. Dr. Feldenkrais discovered that simply attending to body movements with the mind and gaining a more in-depth understanding of how they feel provides opportunities for your body to discover more effective ways of moving. As new ways of moving are learned, your bodymind can more readily adapt to changing needs. I've found moving with awareness to be more effective than traditional stretching for improving both the range and quality of movement.

I think Dr. Feldenkrais would agree that there are no pre-determined right ways for you to move, except that you do so with awareness. The right way is what arises naturally when you attend to whatever movement you are performing. In fact, any exercise can be done mindfully, which can dramatically improve its benefits. I've included the following exercise to assist you as you begin your awareness education:

First, keep in mind and practice what I've written in 2) and 3) above, which will help as you seek to move with awareness. Begin by sitting in a chair and looking over your right shoulder to gauge how far you can see behind you (you may wish to pick an object that represents the limits of your visual field). Now, do the following: keeping your shoulders facing forward, *very slowly and mindfully*, turn your head and neck to the right as far as you can move with minimal effort or exertion. Return to the starting position and repeat ten times. Next, keep your head facing forward while rotating your shoulders to the right, remembering to move slowly and mindfully. Repeat ten times. Finally, combine the two movements, moving head and shoulders together ten times to the right. Afterwards, recheck your range of motion and compare it to what you measured initially. If you're like most people, you significantly exceeded your initial capacity, perhaps to the extent that you're surprised as to how far you're now able to move. If you turn to the left, you will probably notice it remains more restricted and feels different than moving to the right. If you wish, complete the same series of movements to the left and notice the difference.

4) Practicing Mindfulness: Here, I am not referring to minding your manners or your elders (although these aren't bad practices), but maintaining an ongoing awareness of the thoughts, feelings, sensation, and impulses of your bodymind. F.M. Alexander, known for "the Alexander technique," emphasized the importance of being aware of *the way* we do things, rather than simply rushing toward the goal of the activity. For instance, rather than scrambling to finish the dishes, choose to maintain an appreciative awareness of your movements, sensations, and presence as you perform the task.

By practicing mindfulness, you can develop a heightened sensitivity to the needs and desires of your bodymind which can be instrumental in improving your health. Moreover, mindfulness can improve your appreciation and satisfaction with life as a whole, as even the most routine tasks take on new dimension and value. So try it out. Savor your food, savor a shower, savor your work—savor your bodily experiences.

Final Thoughts

In Chapter 4, I suggested that humans possess, on the one hand, amazing potential for self-healing, and on the other, a real capacity for chronic illness. I attribute this largely to factors related to our higher levels of consciousness, which is why animals do not demonstrate the same degree of individual differences when it comes to health.

In my experience, working with bodymind exercises (such as those described above) produces great results. A single session often incorporates the benefits of therapies such as manipulation, stretching, relaxation, and breathwork, as they work together in a unified way. By directing your awareness to your bodily sensations, impulses, feelings, etc., you will discover new avenues of possibility that were previously either ignored or unavailable (This seems true regarding education of any sort, in that the more you know—the more awareness you possess—the more possibilities you begin to see). This type of engagement may reduce your need for clinical assistance, as it allows your bodymind to direct and correct itself.

II

CULTIVATING A POSITIVE OUTLOOK

"Positive Psychology" is a relatively recent but rapidly growing movement within the field of psychology. In cohort with the medical field, psychology has historically focused much of its efforts on describing and treating "abnormality." Those involved with positive psychology, along with advocates of preventative medicine, think there may be a better way of doing things. Specifically, they are interested in identifying and cultivating factors that promote enhanced health and well-being. By discovering what works for healthy people, it may be possible to promote greater public health and reduce the need for clinical intervention.

Hope, optimism, and a positive approach to life are among the many factors known to contribute to well-being (Benson; Brody; Seligman, et al). As discussed in Chapter 4, they are also critical to healing. A positive approach often includes the following characteristics: contentedness, gratefulness (negativity is rooted in focusing on what is missing rather than what is present or possible), a focus on creating solutions rather than dwelling on problems, and embracing optimism as a priority in life.

Some people are more prone to positivity than others. This may be partly genetic, but also has much to do with prior life circumstances and experiences. For instance, extraverts, on average, tend to score higher in optimism than introverts. However, you do not have to be highly outgoing in order to possess a positive, healthy approach to life.

Regardless of your current level of optimism, there is usually room for improvement, should you wish to do so, as a most important factor in cultivating a positive outlook is possessing the will and determination to do so. The remainder of this section will touch on activities and behaviors that can increase positive emotions as well as your sense of engagement with life.

Purpose and meaning are two elements that surface immediately with regard to positivity. Both are generated through multiple means, but often arise out of healthy relationships, the pursuit of personal/community interests and goals, meaningful work, spirituality, etc. Though purpose usually implies action ("My purpose is to..."), meaning can arise from simply appreciating life. One means of cultivating a sense of gratefulness and appreciation is through enhancing your bodily sensitivity and awareness (see Appendix I).

Another way of fostering meaning is through learning and personal development. So often we fool ourselves into believing that we already know what is necessary for optimal living. This can result in a life that seems bland and without further possibility.

Pursuing learning, such as through reading or other forms of exploration, can help you see beyond your current perspective, revealing a world of new perspectives and ideas. Such endeavors can be highly meaningful and may foster a renewed sense of purpose in life. As an example, some of my clients have reported finding renewed meaning in researching their genealogy, sometimes tracing their family lineage back over 500 years. Learning is also helpful for counteracting various misconceptions that may be negatively impacting your health and your life.

The last point I would like to mention is the importance of quality relationships, social support, and job satisfaction in engendering positivity. We all know that it can be difficult to remain positive in an overtly negative and stressful environment. So fostering a more positive approach to life may involve changing or mending your circumstances to provide the necessary space for growth to occur.

You may even discover redirecting your life toward the positive—finding a more meaningful mode of being—to be as valuable as concerted investigation into your pain. In many instances, a positive outlook can nullify the effects of underlying negatives. This again points toward the fact that we are more than a mere aggregation of parts, but function as an orchestrated, integrated whole. We will conclude this section with some final ideas for cultivating a positive outlook (derived from Seligman, et al. Positive Psychotherapy. *American Psychologist.* 774-788. Nov. 2006; www.authentichappiness.org):

- Identify several of your strengths (the above website has a 24-item tool if you need assistance doing so) and find ways to utilize them more regularly.

- In the evening, write down three positive things about your day and why you think they occurred.

- Write about what you would like to be remembered for in your life.

- Compose a letter of gratitude to a person you have never properly thanked.

- Once a day, take time to savor something that you would normally rush through or do without thinking. This may include things such as savoring a meal, enjoying scenery, appreciating bodily sensations while in the shower, moving with heightened awareness, etc.

III

ADDRESSING CHRONIC PAIN & FEAR-AVOIDANCE

John Sarno, a long-time New York physician, is well-known for his alternative approach to treating pain, especially back pain. Dr. Sarno started his career using traditional treatment approaches, such as injections, medications, physical modalities, and other treatments. Wondering why his outcomes were so inconsistent, he began to investigate other variables. His current treatment program is the culmination of several years of observation, questioning, and experimentation.

Dr. Sarno's program focuses on changing the way people conceptualize their pain. After educating his clients about potential sources of their pain, it becomes their responsibility to apply that knowledge to their own situations and change their behavior accordingly. Essentially, his advice involves forsaking the belief that body is damaged or inadequate (e.g. – "I do <u>not</u> have a 'bad back'") and beginning to move and behave in a way consistent with new beliefs. Dr. Sarno has found that if patients can accept and apply his concepts, they get better.

An important part of both Dr. Sarno's and the *Back Sense* programs is using this new understanding of pain toward in overcoming fear-avoidance behavior. Essentially, fear-avoidance is a type of conditioning that involves fearing and avoiding certain activities believed to be associated with pain (see Chapter 5). This is thought to be a primary contributor to both chronicity and disability (Fritz, et al).

In order to overcome this conditioning, you will need to retrain yourself not to fear certain activities by progressively re-engaging in them. During this process, you will learn that your pain is often not a result of the activity itself, but is related to fear, tension, expectations, or other factors. The following suggestions can help you break free of this pain-fear cycle and return to normal activities:

1) Understand what causes pain and repudiate the belief that pain is always a result of a damaged body: Continuously refer to this book (or others like it) as a reminder and resource for this understanding. This will require a disciplined effort to change what may be deeply engrained patterns of thinking. In addition, it is important to relinquish attempts to relieve pain by using gadgets, mattress/shoe changes, or other methods that reinforce the "damaged body" concept.

2) Accept the conditions of recovery:

a) *A full recovery from chronic pain does not usually occur instantaneously:*   Like getting in shape, overcoming fear-avoidance will require persistence and discipline, especially of mind and will.

b) *There will be peaks and valleys to recovery:*   With any painful problem, there will be good days and bad days. If you've struggled with pain for a long time, your road to recovery will be bumpy, often entailing more bad days than good ones early in the process.   Thus, it is important to remain patient and persistent, making sure to notice and celebrate even the smallest improvements.

c) *Focus on function rather than pain:*   When pain is chronic, it is rarely an accurate indicator of bodily damage. So if you are experiencing chronic pain without recent history of a major injury or surgery, it is quite unlikely that pain encountered during activities is indicating that you are damaging your back. It is helpful to recognize your pain as innocuous and stop trying so hard to avoid it. Learning to accept, tolerate, and not fear pain can be challenging and takes time. Enhancing your bodily awareness can assist you in this process (see Appendix I).

3) Set progressive activity goals: Choose an activity that you can perform repeatedly with relative ease and comfort. Over time, increase the speed, duration, frequency, and/or amount of movement. This may involve dividing movements (such as getting out of a chair) into separate components and practicing them individually. Slowly, with practice, you can reintegrate these components until you're successfully performing the complete movement. Awareness through movement exercises (Appendix I) can be useful for improving ease of movement and reducing pain. Walking is another excellent activity for setting progressive, achievable goals.

4) Educate those around you: Often, people who try to help you deal with your pain actually make things worse. By educating them about what you are trying to accomplish, they will be less likely to hinder your progress. Ask them to stop asking about your pain and instead inquire as to how you are doing with your fears and functional goals.

One of the worst aspects of chronic pain is feeling that we must give up beloved activities. This can contribute to dismay and frustration for both you and your loved ones. It is for this reason that working toward returning to normal activities is so critical. With the above strategies (and others described in this book), many people have overcome months and even years of pain and have returned to their prior state of functioning.

IV

BODYMIND CONDITIONS

"All I can say as a scientist is that the great majority of physical illnesses have in part some psychosomatic origin."—Hans Selye, pioneer of stress research

Below is a running list of conditions that may often be driven by factors (described throughout this book) other than medically-described disease processes (see Gatchel & Turk, eds; Sarno; Schlitz & Amorok, eds; Servan-Schreiber, et al; Siegel, et al). In Chapter 2, I described the inconsistent relationship between structural abnormalities and pain. So it is important to remember that even if a bodily structure appears be "abnormal" or "damaged," it may not be a significant contributor to your pain.

- Allergies and asthma (certain types)
- Back/neck pain (often erroneously attributed to degenerative disc disease, herniated discs, arthritis, etc.)
- Cardiopulmonary issues (including various heart-related issues, palpitations, atypical chest pain, hyperventilation)
- Dizziness
- Elbow pain (often erroneously attributed to overuse and labeled tendonitis or tennis elbow)
- Fibromyalgia, chronic fatigue syndrome, myofascial pain syndrome, restless leg, and other pain syndromes
- Foot/heel pain (often erroneously attributed to bone spurs, plantar fascitis, flat arches, or tendonitis)
- Headaches
- High blood pressure/hypertension
- Hip pain (sometimes erroneously attributed to arthritis or bursitis)
- Gastrointestinal symptoms (stomach discomfort, nausea, irritable bowel syndrome, gastric reflux, ulcers, etc.)
- Knee pain (often erroneously attributed to meniscus/cartilage tears, problems involving the knee cap, or arthritis)
- Pseudoneurologic symptoms (ringing in the ears/tinnitus, blurred vision, fainting, pseudoseizures, muscle weakness, etc.)
- Shoulder pain (often erroneously attributed to tendonitis, bursitis or rotator cuff damage)
- Sleep/sexual/menstrual problems
- TMJ (jaw pain/clicking)
- Various skin disorders
- Wrist pain (often erroneously attributed to carpal tunnel syndrome)
- Other disorders

Pain always involves the whole person—mind, body, emotions, environment, culture, relationships, etc. So attempt to distinguish "medical disease" from other bodymind disorders is problematic, as *all* health conditions are situated within a certain context of influence. That notwithstanding, I decided to include the above list to help us look beneath or beyond a given diagnosis. In other words, many of the above share common origins in an imbalanced bodymind and will benefit from the application of the information in this book.

Diagnoses Associated with Back/Neck Pain

As a practicing physical therapist, it was not long before I was struck by the prevalence of back and neck pain in our culture. In fact, these problems were largely responsible for piquing my interest in the subject of pain. So I wanted to briefly comment on a few of the more common diagnoses and how they are related to pain.

Degenerative Disc Disease (DDD): DDD entails a flattening of spinal discs which occurs as they lose their ability to retain fluid over time. Rarely is DDD alone a significant contributor to pain, although exceptions can probably be found in the elderly population.

Bulging/Ruptured/Herniated Disc: A tear/rupture of a spinal disc can lead to acute back pain, but rarely does it cause chronic problems (an exception may be a disc impinging on the spinal cord). This diagnosis is used far too often as an explanation for persistent back and neck pain. While it is true that severe or recent disc herniations may contribute to symptoms such as pain, tingling, numbness, burning, and weakness in the leg, we also know that many people with disc herniations experience absolutely no pain (Gatchel & Turk, eds; Jensen, et al; Borenstein, et al). Therefore, in most cases, conservative treatment, including ideas presented in this book, should be thoroughly exhausted prior to any invasive intervention (there may be exceptions for severe injuries).

"Pinched Nerve"/Sciatica: Deriving its name from the major nerve that innervates the lower extremities (i.e., the sciatic nerve; there are actually two of them), sciatica generally refers to pain (or other undesirable symptoms) that radiates from the low back or buttock region into the hip/thigh/leg (this may also be referred to as radiculopathy). As discussed in Chapter 5, radiating pain is often attributed to a "pinched nerve," rather than more appropriately to chemical irritation (such as from inflammation) or other factors described in this book. Despite its sometimes sharp, shooting nature, sciatica, like other types of pain, is usually benign, making it fully amenable to the management strategies described in this book.

"Subluxation"/"Out of Alignment": As discussed in previously, viewing the body as merely a machine is inadequate in light of the current evidence. Often, chiropractic treatments provide only temporary relief when joints are released of surrounding tension. The lack of lasting relief may be due to the fact that tension depends on multiple factors such as posturing, motor patterns/programs, psychoemotional factors, etc. Consequently, recurring patterns of tension often return within minutes or hours of treatment. This is not to say that these treatments never produce long-term relief, since small changes in the bodymind may lead to disproportionate changes in the whole. Most chiropractic, however, is not holistic (even if marketed as such), but tends to reinforce the body-machine concept and engender overdependence on "quick-fix" treatments.

V

CLINICAL CONSIDERATIONS

Many researchers and clinicians make a point of differentiating between acute and chronic pain. Acute pain refers to that which is fairly recent in onset, whereas chronic pain is typically that which endures longer than three months. In many instances, this is a useful method of classification.

Following an injury, for example, the prescription of a few days rest and passive treatments, such as icing or anti-inflammatory medication, is often beneficial. However, passive treatments become significantly less effective as time transpires. So when managing chronic pain, the focus should entail more active strategies.

Despite its clinical utility, the acute-chronic dichotomy can be misapplied and misleading in many cases of pain. This misapplication occurs primarily with those individuals whose pain is related to psychosomatic processes. Here is an example:

Becky, only 43 years old, feels that her body is falling apart. She has now undergone seven surgeries, each performed in a different area of her body. She presents with a growing list of diagnoses and is taking numerous prescription drugs. After waking up with terrific neck pain without known injury, she visits a surgeon who orders an MRI. The MRI indicates a slight bulging disc which he suggests as a potential cause of the problem. Becky cannot believe that she may require yet another surgery and feels helpless with respect to her ongoing difficulties. She attributes her problems to having been dealt a defective body and concludes that she will probably suffer the consequences the rest of her life.

In this common scenario, Becky would not necessarily have been classified as having "chronic pain," since her neck pain had begun just recently. The physician, perhaps slow to connect the emerging pattern of painful problems, continued to view her pain from a body-machine perspective. This would appear especially likely if her prior surgeries were reported to have been "successful." After all, if her other painful problems had abated with treatment, chances are that history would repeat itself and she would be satisfied, at least temporarily.

In situations such as these, treatment may provide temporary relief of symptoms, which may be largely attributable to the placebo effect (see Chapter 4). However, the pain often returns under a different guise, perhaps moving from a recently treated shoulder to the knee or low back. In Appendix IV, I included a list of conditions that are often believed to be related to tissue damage but may actually be resulting from other factors described in this book. So what is diagnosed as "tendonitis," for instance, may merely be a manifestation of a more comprehensive state of bodymind imbalance.

I refer to pain that is not chronically present in a single area but manifests at different bodily sites over time as "recurrent pain." As described above, individuals experiencing recurrent pain may often respond to treatment, only to return with a different symptom following a short respite. In Chapter 5, I discussed the importance of attempting to identify root causes of pain. This appears especially critical with respect to recurrent pain, as conventional approaches are not actually solving the problem, but merely administering a temporary patch.

Management strategies will be very similar for recurrent and chronic pain. Both types will be best served by a multifaceted approach, such as that described in this book. In many cases, recurrent pain is actually easier to treat and may also be more amenable to permanent eradication.

Diagnosis

The process of diagnosis should involve attempting to identify foundational sources of the problem (see Chapter 5). The following points pertain to clinical diagnosis of patients reporting pain:

- In the absence of recent injury, most cases of back or neck pain will involve significant contributions from psychosocial factors, muscle tension, and/or movement dysfunction. Other important factors to consider are age, gender, socioeconomic status, relationship issues/social support, sexual/substance abuse, prior trauma, pain in other body parts, and history of psychological issues and/or bodymind conditions (see list in Appendix IV). Those with multiple medical problems or complicating factors, such as obesity or diabetes, are more susceptible to pain as a result of unfavorable physiological conditions.

- Pain reported by patients receiving worker's compensation and those of lower socioeconomic status may involve a myriad of psychosocial stressors and related muscle tension. Even if an injury was purported to be involved, research suggests that psychosocial factors and related behaviors play a central role in the progression to chronicity and disability (Bigos, et al; Gatchel & Turk, eds; Williams, et al; Pincus, et al).

- The first six weeks following an onset of pain are critical for preventing chronicity and addressing fear-avoidance behavior (Fritz, et al).

- Ask the patient if anything has changed within the past year or so that could be interpreted as stressful. Has (s)he been recently widowed, divorced, lost a job, etc. These stressors can powerfully contribute to crossing the bodymind's pain threshold.

- Observation: Does the patient seem angry, stressed, anxious, depressed, pessimistic, or have difficulty relaxing? Does (s)he gravitate toward worst-case scenarios (i.e., catastrophize), worrying that (s)he will never get better, or does (s)he seem to cope well?

- For a look at some of the criteria for diagnosing psychosomatic conditions, clinicians may wish to review information pertaining to somatization and somatoform disorders (see Servan-Schreibner, et al. for a good introduction). The term somatization is sometimes given slightly different definitions, but generally describes a process by which psychoemotional distress manifests as physical symptoms. Somatoform disorders are specific psychiatric diagnoses (see DSM-IV) which include somatization disorder (a more specific classification than "somatization"), pain disorder, conversion disorder, and undifferentiated somatoform disorder. Though I do not believe these formal diagnostic criteria are all that helpful, it has been suggested that providing patients with a diagnosis can be more helpful than not doing so (Servan-Schreiber, et al). Somatization may be a useful descriptor, in that it has not acquired the negative connotations of the pithier "psychosomatic."

Strategies for Assisting Patients in Pain

Appropriate treatment for patients presenting with significant psychoemotional contributions can range from fairly simple to complex. As most clinicians have already discovered, the most difficult patients to treat are those with chronic pain, multiple medical problems, low educational/socioeconomic status, worker's compensation status, a history of psychological disorders, a history of abuse/trauma, substance abusers, etc. For difficult cases of chronic pain, inpatient interdisciplinary pain management programs may be the most efficacious and cost-effective treatment (Gatchel). More generally, patients may benefit from the following:

- *Education about Pain*: If you run short on time in the clinic, you might consider group educational sessions and/or the use of media, such as handouts or educational videos.

- *A Quality Therapeutic Relationship*: Attempt to balance an empathetic, listening ear with sound advice.

- *Healing Communication*: This involves recognizing the power of words and manner to activate the patient's self-healing capabilities (see Chapter 4).

- *Restoration of Movement*: Encourage movement of the painful area and returning to normal daily activities, including work, even in the presence of some pain. This will need to be buttressed with pain education, being sure to emphasize the fact that increasing physical activity will not be harmful. For more recent onsets of pain, returning to activity may be abetted by short-term use of medications or other modalities.

- *Integrated/Bodymind Therapies*: Meditation, yoga, tai-chi, biofeedback, Feldenkrais, hypnosis, body psychotherapy, etc.

- *Judicious Use of Specialists and Passive Modalities*: Specialists do just that—specialize—and are prone to be less likely to consider the bigger picture. Over-utilization of outside referrals, as well as frequent use of passive modalities, risks unwanted reinforcement of a myopic understanding of pain.

- *Community Assistance/Involvement*: Social work, career/ vocational counseling, psychotherapy, support groups, etc.

VI

PAIN, STRESS, & PHYSIOLOGY

"All sensory phenomena, including nocioception, can be altered by conscious or unconscious mental processes."—John D. Louser, "What is Chronic Pain?" *Theoretical Medicine* 12(3): 214-15. 1991.

The International Association for the Study of Pain (IASP) defines pain as: *"An unpleasant sensory and emotional experience associated with actual or potential tissue damage, or described in terms of such damage."* The IASP subcommittee added the following: *"Activity induced in the nocioceptor...is not pain, which is always a psychological state."*

In other words, the world's leading panel of experts on pain is no longer conceptualizing pain as a mere sensation indicating tissue damage, but is now heralding the importance of emotional and psychological factors.

A concise and understandable explanation of the physiological connections between stress, pain, and illness has been offered by renowned pain researcher Dr. Robert Melzack (he and Patrick Wall pioneered the "Gate Theory of Pain") in his contribution to *Psychosocial Factors in Pain.* Here, I will provide an overview of Melzack's synthesis.

First, Melzack asserts: *"Pain...is produced by the output of a widely distributed neural network... rather than directly by sensory input evoked by injury, inflammation, or other pathology."* He refers to this network as the "neuromatrix" whose output is *"determined by multiple influences, of which somatic sensory input is only a part"* (I have emphasized this throughout the book).

Melzack goes on to discuss stress: *"The disruption of homeostasis by a stressor, either physical or psychological, activates programs of neural, hormonal, and behavioral activity aimed at restoring homeostasis."* These concepts should sound familiar to the rhetoric used throughout this book, only that I chose to use the more user-friendly term "balance" in place of "homeostasis." Melzack proceeds to posit four systems that he calls *"stress-regulation programs,"* which serve to restore homeostasis:

1) Hypothalamic-Pituitary-Adrenal (HPA) System: Activation of this system, either through psychological stress or physical injury, eventually results in cortisol being released into the bloodstream. Cortisol has the potential to be highly destructive, as it can break down muscle protein and inhibit calcium resorption into bone. Melzack indicates that the destructive effects of cortisol on the body may make injury more likely (including repeated minor injuries), which could eventually contribute to pain.

2) Sympathetic Nervous System: All medical professionals should be familiar with this system, as well as its effects on heart rate, respiration, blood pressure, and muscle tone. This system is typically predominant in those with chronic stress or anxiety, and is sometimes evidenced by faster/shallower breathing, heightened muscle tone, etc. It is important to note that hormones associated with the sympathetic response have been shown to exacerbate neural irritation and pain (Butler).

3) Immune System: In Chapter 5, I described the contribution of inflammation—a product of the immune system—to pain. Another germane issue is the suppression of the immune system during times of significant stress. According to Humphrey (2002), such immune suppression may be rooted in the redistribution of bodily resources according to one's expectations.

For instance, if I am being chased by a lion, my foremost need is high levels adrenaline to avoid becoming Leo's lunch. This means that other processes, such as immunity or digestion, must be temporarily set aside in order to mobilize resources for imminent survival needs. The take home point is when immune functioning is suppressed via stress or other means, we are at greater risk of encountering pain or illness. In some cases, the immune system rebounds and attacks itself, leading to a variety of autoimmune diseases.

4) Limbic-Cortical Interaction System: This may be the most important of the stress systems with regard to pain. Melzack writes,

"*The limbic system...is the affective-motivational dimension of pain and a portion of (it), including the hypothalamus, is an integral part of the stress system. The two systems are so interdependent that they should be considered as components of a single system.*" With Melzack, the relationship between stress, emotions, and pain, has comprised a central feature of this book.0

Additional Thoughts

In addition to Melzack, we should not overlook the contribution of the central nervous system to chronic pain, as morphological changes in the spinal cord and/or brain may amplify peripheral nociceptive signals. An overview is provided in David Butler's *The Sensitive Nervous System*, which nicely describes both central and peripheral neurobiological processes related to nocioception.

Dr. Candace Pert also makes important contributions to our scientific groundwork in her book *Molecules of Emotion*. Pert, who spearheaded pioneering research into neuropeptides, has explicated the physiology of emotions, including the process of ligand-receptor binding. Such binding occurs both peripherally and in the brain, influencing not only the state of individual cells, but the conscious experience of the whole organism. Thus, according to Pert, neuropeptides serve as a critical bridge between "mind" and "body."

RECOMMENDED READING

For General Readership:

Back Sense, by Ronald Siegel, Michael Urdang, and Douglas Johnson: An excellent example of a self pain-management program, including extensive references, activities, and additional resources.

The Mindbody Prescription, by John Sarno: As mentioned previously, John Sarno is a pioneer in mind-body medicine, especially in the treatment of back pain. He is the author of numerous books.

Timeless Healing, by Herbert Benson: A valuable and comprehendible resource, written by a respected Harvard physician and researcher.

For Those in Health-Related Professions:

Clinical Essentials of Pain Management, by Robert Gatchel: Written by a foremost pain researcher, this reasonably priced resource is a good place to start for any clinician. It provides a broad overview for the understanding, assessment, and management of pain. Included are many useful figures summarizing essential concepts, diagnostic tests, treatments, etc. At the end of each chapter are appendices which display helpful examples and assist with application.

Psychosocial Factors in Pain, edited by Robert Gatchel and Dennis Turk: This is a wonderful compilation of peer-reviewed research that compellingly demonstrates the powerful interactions of mind, body, and environment with respect to pain. The research discussed serves to elucidate why and how the "biopsychosocial model" is critical to understanding and managing pain and illness. This is an important reference for any professional regularly treating or researching painful conditions.

Consciousness & Healing, Marilyn Schlitz and Tina Amorok with Marc Micozzi: Full of valuable insights, interesting research, and progressive thinking about the future of medicine, this thought provoking anthology, containing over 60 essays, skillfully negotiates the tenuous philosophical spectrums of reductionism-idealism, empiricism-holism, and modernism-postmodernism.

The Sensitive Nervous System, by David Butler: This book was written primarily for physical therapists. In fact, it was the volume from which I gained my introduction to thinking about pain in its broader contexts. Butler presents current neurobiological concepts of pain while maintaining due respect for relevant psychosocial factors. Though I found this book most helpful for its theoretical foundations, Butler provides applicable clinical suggestions as well. This is easily among the most helpful and scientifically-grounded references for physical therapists who regularly assist people in pain.

The Renewal of Generosity, by Arthur Frank: This book embodies a moral call to all who participate in caring for others. Frank espouses that clinicians are generous when they attempt to understand patients as they are and assist them in providing clarity to their experiences. Frank's complex interweaving of stories and reflections resists reduction into a formula for practicing medicine, but helps caregivers remember and enhance the overarching purpose of their work.

The Human Effect in Medicine, by Michael Dixon and Karen Sweeney: This book nicely summarizes the current evidence base for the placebo or "human effect." It also offers practical ideas for nurturing the human effect in the clinic, along with detailed documentation of references.

Imagery in Healing, by Jeanne Achterberg: Highly recommended. Achterberg is a scientist-practitioner and erudite writer who integrates much of her own research with that of several related disciplines. For those who enjoy a balanced exploration of the historical, psychological, philosophical, and physiological aspects of the mind in healing, this is an excellent choice.

Rethinking Psychiatry, by Arthur Kleinman: Any of Arthur Kleinman's books, though academic in nature, are excellent for gaining an understanding of the prominent role of culture in illness and healing. I especially liked this one.

SOURCES

Achterberg J. *Imagery in Healing.* Boston: Shambhala. 1985.

Aposhyan S. *Natural Intelligence: Body-Mind Integration and Human Development.* Lippincott Williams & Wilkins. 1999.

Arraj J. *Tracking the Elusive Human Volume II: An Advanced Guide to the Typological Worlds of C.G Jung, W.H. Sheldon, Their Integration, and the Biochemical Typology of the Future.* Chiloquin, OR: Inner Growth Books. 1990.

Bayer T, Baer P, & Charles E. Situational and Psychophysiological Factors in Psychologically Induced Pain. *Pain.* 44(1):45-50. 1991.

Benson H. *Timeless Healing: The Power and Biology of Belief.* New York: Scribner. 1996.

Bigos SJ, et al. A Prospective Study of Work Perceptions and Psychosocial Factors Affecting the Reporting of a Back Injury. *Spine.* 16(1):1-6. 1991.

Boddeker I & Stemmler G. Who Responds How and When to Anger? The Assessment of Actual Anger Response Styles and Their Relation to Personality. *Cognition and Emotion.* 14(6):737-62. 2000.

Bogduk N. Management of Chronic Low Back Pain. *Medical Journal of Australia.* 180(2):79-83. 2004.

Sources

Borenstein DG, et al. The Value of Magnetic Resonance Imaging of the Lumbar Spine to Predict Low-Back Pain in Asymptomatic Subjects. *The Journal of Bone and Joint Surgery.* 83-A(9):1306-11. 2001.

Brena SF, Sanders SH, & Motoyama H. American and Japanese Low Back Pain Patients: Cross-Cultural Similarities and Differences. *Clinical Journal of Pain.* 6(2):118-24. 1990.

Brody H. *The Placebo Response: How You Can Release the Body's Inner Pharmacy for Better Health.* New York: Harper Collins. 2000.

Bru E. The Role of Psychological Factors in Neck, Shoulder, and Low Back Pain among Female Hospital Staff. *Rogaland Research.* Stravenger, Norway. 1994.

Butler D. *The Sensitive Nervous System.* Adelaide: Noigroup Publications. 2000.

Carron H, DeGood D, & Tait R. A Comparison of Low Back Pain Patients in the United States and New Zealand: Psychological and Economic Factors Affecting Severity and Disability. *Pain.* 21(1):77-89. 1985.

Chatterjee C. Stop the Pain. *Psychology Today.* Sep-Oct, 1999.

Claxton G. *The Wayward Mind: An Intimate History of the Unconscious.* London: Abacus. 2005.

Cole S, et al. Elevated Physical Health Risk among Gay Men Who Conceal Their Homosexual Identity. *Health Psychology.* 15(4):243-51. 1996.

Sources

Cousins N. *Anatomy of an Illness as Perceived by the Patient: Reflections on Healing and Regeneration.* W.W. Norton & Company. 2001.

Cymet TC & Sinkov V. Does Long-Distance Running Cause Osteoarthritis? *The Journal of the American Osteopathic Association.* 106(6):342-45. 2006.

Dimond EG, Kittle CF, & Crockett JE. Comparison of Internal Mammary Ligation and Sham Operation for Angina Pectoris. *American Journal of Cardiology.* 5:483-86. 1960.

Dixon M & Sweeney K. *The Human Effect in Medicine: Theory, Research, and Practice.* Abingdon: Radcliffe Medical Press. 2000.

Dossey L. *Reinventing Medicine.* San Francisco: Harper Collins. 1999.

Dychtwald K. *Bodymind.* New York: Penguin Putnam. 1986.

Feldenkrais M. *The Elusive Obvious.* Capitola, CA: Meta Publications. 1981.

Fink DH. *Release from Nervous Tension.* New York: Pocket Books. 1962.

Fox AJ, et al. Myelographic Cervical Nerve Root Deformities. *Radiology.* 116:355-61. 1975.

Frank AW. *The Renewal of Generosity: Illness, Medicine, and How to Live.* Chicago: University of Chicago Press. 2004.

Sources

Frankl V. *Man's Search for Meaning: An Introduction to Logotherapy.* New York: Simon & Schuster. 1984.

Fries JF, et al. Running and the Development of Disability with Age. *Annals of Internal Medicine.* 121:502-509. 1994.

Fritz JM, George SZ, & Delito A. The Role of Fear-Avoidance Beliefs in Acute Low Back Pain: Relationships with Current and Future Disability and Work Status. *Pain.* 92:7-13. 2001.

Gatchel RJ. *Clinical Essentials of Pain Management.* Washington: American Psychological Association. 2005.

Gatchel RJ & Turk DC, eds. *Psychosocial Factors in Pain: Critical Perspectives.* New York: Guilford Publications. 1999.

Ghaly M & Telplitz D. The Biologic Effects of Grounding the Human Body During Sleep by Cortisol Levels and Subjective Reports of Sleep, Pain, and Stress. *Journal of Alternative and Complementary Medicine.* 10(5):767-76. 2004.

Gladwell M. *Blink: The Power of Thinking Without Thinking.* New York: Time Warner. 2005.

Gottfredson LS. Intelligence: Is It the Epidemiologists' Elusive "Fundamental Cause" of Social Class Inequalities in Health? *Journal of Personality and Social Psychology.* 86(1):174-79. 2004.

Sources

Hall E & Haydel M. Conversion Disorder Presenting as Hemiplegia and Hemianesthesia with Loss of Neurologic Reflexes: A Case Report. *Southern Medical Journal.* 99(4):380-2. 2006.

Hardcastle VG. *The Myth of Pain.* Massachusetts Institute of Technology. 1999.

Houston J. *Life Force: The Psycho-Historical Recovery of the Self.* Wheaton: The Theosophical Publishing House. 1993.

Humphrey N. Great Expectations: The Evolutionary Psychology of Faith-Healing and the Placebo Response. In *Psychology at the Turn of the Millenium, Vol. 2.* von Hofsten C & Backman L, eds. Hove: Psychology Press. 2002.

Illich I. *Medical Nemesis: The Expropriation of Health.* Random House. 1976.

Kepner J. *Body Process: Working with the Body in Psychotherapy.* San Francisco: Jossey-Bass Publishers. 1987.

Kleinman A. *Rethinking Psychiatry.* New York: MacMillan. 1988.

Kosambi DD. Living Prehistory in India. *Scientific American.* 216:105-14. 1967.

Kroenke K, Arrington ME, & Mangelsdorff AD. The Prevalence of Symptoms in Medical Outpatients and the Adequacy of Therapy. *Archives of Internal Medicine.* 150:1685-90. 1990.

Sources

Jensen MC, et al. Magnetic Resonance Imaging of the Lumbar Spine in People without Back Pain. *New England Journal of Medicine.* 331(2):69-73. 1994.

Levine P. *Waking the Tiger: Healing Trauma.* Berkeley: North Atlantic Books. 1997.

Lipton B. *The Biology of Belief.* Santa Rosa: Elite Books. 2005.

Lounsbury JW, et al. Personality, Career Satisfaction, and Life Satisfaction. *Journal of Career Assessment.* 12(4):395-406. 2004.

Louser JD. Low Back Pain. In *Pain*, ed. Borice JJ. *Research Publications: Association for Research in Nervous and Mental Disease.* 58:363-77. New York: Raven. 1980.

Lucire Y. Neurosis in the Workplace. *Medical Journal of Austrailia.* 145:323-27. 1986.

Martin P. *The Healing Mind.* New York: St. Martin's Press. 1997.

Macnaughton I. *Body, Breath, & Consciousness: A Somatics Anthology.* Berkeley: North Atlantic Books. 2004.

Melzack R, Wall PD, & Ty TC. Acute Pain in an Emergency Clinic: Latency of Onset and Descriptor Patterns Related to Different Injuries. *Pain.* 14:33-43.

Morris D. *Illness and Culture in the Postmodern Age.* Berkeley: University of California Press. 1998.

Sources

Moseley B, et al. A Controlled Trial of Arthroscopic Surgery for Osteoarthritis of the Knee. *New England Journal of Medicine.* 347(2):81-88. 2002.

Nathan B. *Touch and Emotion in Manual Therapy.* London: Churchill Livingstone. 1999.

Newth S & Delongis A. Individual Differences, Mood, and Coping with Chronic Pain in Rheumatoid Arthritis: A Daily Process Analysis. *Psychology and Health.* 19:283-305. 2004.

Nicklas BJ, You T, & Pahor M. Behavioral Treatment for Chronic Systemic Inflammation: Effects of Dietary Weight Loss and Exercise. *Canadian Medical Association Journal.* 172(9):1199-1209.

Ornish D. *Love and Survival: The Scientific Basis for the Healing Power of Intimacy.* New York: HarperCollins. 1998.

Payer L. *Culture and Medicine.* United States: Henry Holt. 1988.

Pengel LHM, et al. Acute Low Back Pain: Systematic Review of Its Prognosis. *The British Medical Journal.* 327:323-27. 2003.

Pennebaker JW. Confession, Inhibition, and Disease. *Adv Exp Soc Psych.* 22:212-44. 1989.

Pert C. *Molecules of Emotion.* New York: Scribner. 1997.

Pincus T, et al. A Systematic Review of Psychological Factors as Predictors of Chronicity/Disability in Prospective Cohorts of Low Back Pain. *Spine.* 27(5):E109-E120. 2002.

Prinz P. Sleep, Appetite, and Obesity—What is the Link? *PLoS Med.* 1(3):e61.

Roter, et al. Effectiveness of Interventions to Improve Patient Compliance: A Meta-Analysis. *Medical Care.* 36:1138-61. 1998.

Sanders SH, et al. Chronic Low Back Pain Patients around the World: Cross Cultural Similarities and Differences. *Clinical Journal of Pain.* 8(4):317-23. 1992.

Sapolsky RM. *Why Zebras Don't Get Ulcers: An Updated Guide to Stress, Stress-Related Diseases, and Coping.* New York: W.H. Freeman. 1998.

Sarno J. *The Mindbody Prescription: Healing the Body, Healing the Pain.* New York: Warner Books. 1998.

Scarry E. *The Body in Pain: The Making and Unmaking of the World.* New York: Oxford University Press. 1985.

Schlitz M & Amorok T, eds. *Consciousness and Healing: Integral Approaches to Mind-Body Medicine.* St. Louis: Churchill-Livingston. 2005.

Seligman MEP, Rashid T, & Parks AC. Positive Psychotherapy. *American Psychologist.* 774-788. Nov. 2006.

Sources

Servan-Schreiber D, Kolb NR, & Tabas G. Somatizing Patients: Part I. Practical Diagnosis. *American Family Physician.* 61:1073-78. 2000.

Shrader H, et al. Natural Evolution of Late Whiplash Syndrome Outside the Medicolegal Context. *Lancet.* 347(9010):1207-11. 1996.

Shutty MS, et al. Chronic Pain Patient's Beliefs about Their Pain and Treatment Outcomes. *Archives of Physical Medicine and Rehabilitation.* 71(2):128-32. 1990.

Siegel BS. *Love, Medicine, & Miracles: Lessons Learned about Self-Healing from a Surgeon's Experience with Exceptional Patients.* New York: Harper & Row. 1986.

Siegel RD, Urdang MH, & Johnson DR. *Back Sense: A Revolutionary Approach to Halting the Cycle of Chronic Back Pain.* New York: Broadway Books. 2001.

Smith AP. *The Power of Thought to Heal: An Ontology of Personal Faith.* Dissertation. Claremont Graduate University. 1998.

Smolkin MT. *Understanding Pain: Interpretation and Philosophy.* Malabar: Krieger Publishing. 1989.

Spangforte EV. The Lumbar Disk Herniation: A Computer-Aided Analysis of 2504 Operations. *Acta Orthopaedica Scandinavica.* 142:1-95. 1972.

Spiegal D, et al. Effect of Psychosocial Treatment on Survival of Patients with Metastatic Breast Cancer. *Lancet.* 2:888-91. 1989.

Sources

Symonds TL, et al. Absence Resulting from Low Back Trouble Can Be Reduced by Psychosocial Intervention at the Work Place. *Spine.* 20(24):2738-45. 1995.

Szabo RM & King KJ. Repetitive Stress Injury: Diagnosis or Self-Fulfilling Prophecy? *The Journal of Bone and Joint Surgery.* 82A:1314-22. 2000.

Waddell G. *The Back Pain Revolution.* Edinburgh: Churchill Livingstone. 1998.

Wall PD. *Pain: The Science of Suffering.* London: Weidenfeld & Nicholson. 1999.

Wilber K. *Integral Psychology: Consciousness, Spirit, Psychology, Therapy.* Boston: Shambhala. 2000.

Williams RA, et al. The Contribution of Job Satisfaction to the Transition from Acute to Chronic Low Back Pain. *Archives of Physical Medicine and Rehabilitation.* 79:366-73. 1998.

INDEX

A

acute pain, 141
anger, 79
ankle pain, 57
anti-depressants, 22
anti-inflammatory medication, 63
anxiety, 29, 53, 75, 76, 77, 78, 107,
    149
arthritis, 19, 40, 62, 63, 138
awareness, bodily, 27, 51, 52, 53, 74,
    75, 80, 84, 86, 89, 104, 124, 125,
    126, 127, 128, 130, 135, 136

B

back pain, 12, 14, 18, 19, 20, 21, 22,
    30, 36, 42, 43, 44, 45, 51, 56, 59,
    62, 67, 72, 76, 105, 131, 133, 134,
    135, 138, 139, 140, 143, 151
    surgery, 22
balance, 27-33, 46, 56, 96, 97, 102,
    104, 106, 115, 125, 142, 148
biofeedback, 37, 146
body chemistry, 51, 61, 63, 140
body weight, 60, 105
body-machine, 13, 14, 15, 19, 58, 60,
    63, 64, 66, 70, 103, 119, 140, 142
bodymind, 7, 20, 26, 27, 28, 29, 30,
    31, 33, 36, 46, 50, 52, 53, 54, 56,
    67, 70, 74, 75, 76, 78, 84, 86, 87,
    96, 98, 102, 104, 106, 107, 114,
    115, 125, 126, 127, 130, 135, 137,
    139, 140, 143, 144
bodywork, 51, 53, 88, 109
bone spurs, 14, 19, 138
bursitis, 138
Butler, David, 149, 150, 152

C

cancer, 37, 62, 81, 88
cardiovascular disease, 62, 79, 81,
    138
carpal tunnel syndrome, 14, 51, 64,
    138
cartilage tears, 19, 138
CEO acronym, 8, 47, 103
ceremonial healing, 46
chiropractic, 106, 140
chronic fatigue syndrome, 138
chronic pain, 1, 2, 4, 5, 57, 59, 62,
    94, 95, 97, 108, 135, 136, 141,
    142, 143, 145, 150
context, of pain, 3, 10, 29, 92, 101,
    106
conversion disorder, 35, 145
culture, role in pain, 12, 13, 21, 31,
    60, 70, 80, 119, 153

D

degenerative disc disease, 139
depression, 35, 45, 51, 59, 61, 67, 78
diagnosis, 19, 37, 39, 60, 118, 139,
    143
diaphragmatic breathing, 76
diet, 27, 61, 62, 77
disability, 20, 42, 56, 64, 65, 118,
    134, 144
dizziness, 138
dysfunctional altruism, 71

E

elbow pain, 138
emotions, 15, 16, 22, 23, 67, 79, 80,
    81, 83, 84, 85, 86, 87, 88, 89, 103,
    104, 106, 130, 150
    repression, 85, 86

Index

P

perfectionism, 71, 79
personality, 20, 51, 71, 77, 79, 80, 124
Pert, Candace, 84, 114, 150, 161
phantom pain, 3
physical therapy, 22, 39, 65, 139
pinched nerve, 62, 140
placebo effect, 22, 39, 40, 41
sham surgery, 22
plantar fascitis, 138
posture, 51, 65, 66, 67, 108
psychotherapy, 87, 146
purpose, 61, 78, 84, 92, 93, 94, 97, 130, 131

R

Reich, Wilhem, 97
relaxation, 54, 74, 76, 107, 125
restless leg syndrome, 138
rolfing, 51, 52
rotator cuff, 14, 19, 138

S

Sarno, John, 46, 86, 87, 119, 133, 151
sciatica, 140
self-fulfilling prophecy, 38, 39, 40, 117
self-healing, 33
shoulder pain, 14, 138

sleep, 72, 76
social support, 81
socioeconomic status, 70, 144, 145
somatization, 144
somatoform disorders, 144
stress, 15, 30, 44, 50, 53, 59, 61, 63, 65, 72, 73, 74, 75, 76, 77, 78, 79, 80, 86, 98, 99, 104, 106, 115, 118, 148, 149
management strategies, 73
subconscious, 50, 80, 84, 86, 87, 111
subluxation, 140
suffering, 22, 91, 92, 94, 99
sympathetic nervous system, 149

T

tendonitis, 51, 64, 65, 138, 142
tension, 20, 44, 45, 50, 52, 53, 54, 61, 75, 78, 85, 86, 104, 107, 125, 134, 140, 143, 144
threshold, pain/bodymind, 28, 29, 30, 52, 72, 85, 104, 115, 144
tinnitus, 138
TMJ, 138
trauma, 50, 73, 86, 143, 145

W

Wall, Patrick, 28, 148
wear and tear myth, 64
whiplash, 21
white coat prophecy, 39
Wilber, Ken, 34, 164
wrist pain, 14, 64, 138

167

PERSONAL AND ONLINE CONSULTATIONS
WITH THE AUTHOR

Re-Thinking Pain addresses why and how pain should be understood in its life contexts. If the context of your pain is not considered, as is commonly practiced in healthcare, it is more likely to continue unabated. Because of the importance of life circumstances, as well as how you think and behave toward pain, fancy equipment and special testing are often unnecessary. Instead, pain can be significantly reduced through the means of education, dialogue, and guidance. With this in mind, Drew has opted to make himself available for face-to-face as well as online consultations. Online consulting has many benefits including personal convenience, reduced cost, and the ease of preserving important dialogue and advice. If you are interested in working with Drew, please feel free to e-mail him:

drew@rethinkpain.com

You may also wish to visit his website, www.rethinkpain.com, for additional information on consultations, upcoming presentations, and other services, or to purchase additional copies of this book.

Give Re-Thinking Pain to
Your Friends & Colleagues

To order online using credit or debit through Paypal visit:

www.rethinkpain.com

(discounts may be available with online orders)

-or-

Send this form, along with a check or money order for $14.95 + $2.99 shipping and handling per book to:

Drew Drenth
54203 Stonebridge Drive
Elkhart, IN 46514

_____ Specify the number of copies you are requesting.

Please e-mail the author with any comments about how this book has helped you or someone you know:

drew@rethinkpain.com